Emerging Leaders in Academic Medicine

Arjang Djamali • Fahad Aziz • Dana Clark

Emerging Leaders in Academic Medicine

A Concise Guide to Navigating the Path to Leadership Success

Springer

Arjang Djamali
Medicine
Maine Medical Center, MaineHealth
Portland, ME, USA

Fahad Aziz
Nephrology
University of Wisconsin Hospital
and Clinics
Madison, WI, USA

Dana Clark
Academic Affairs
MaineHealth
Portland, ME, USA

ISBN 978-3-031-80360-4 ISBN 978-3-031-80358-1 (eBook)
https://doi.org/10.1007/978-3-031-80358-1

Editorial Contact: Richard Lansing
This Springer imprint is published by the registered company Springer Nature Switzerland AG
The registered company address is: Gewerbestrasse 11, 6330 Cham, Switzerland

Introduction

In the fast-paced and dynamic environment of academic medicine, leaders are crucial to driving innovation, fostering collaboration, and advancing the field to new heights. For early-stage physicians embarking on their academic careers, the journey to becoming effective leaders can be both challenging and rewarding. This book, *Emerging Leaders in Academic Medicine: A Concise Guide to Navigating the Path to Leadership*, is designed as a guide for aspiring academic leaders as they navigate the complexities of leadership, unlock their potential, and achieve success in their careers.

Chapter 1: Who Am I, and Who Do I Want to Be?. The first step in the journey to academic leadership is self-discovery. In this chapter, we delve into the fundamental questions of identity and purpose that shape our leadership journey. By exploring our values, strengths, and aspirations, we lay the foundation for authentic and effective leadership. Through introspection and self-assessment, early-stage physicians can gain clarity on their personal and professional identities, setting the stage for intentional growth and development as leaders in academic medicine.

Chapter 2: Starting Your New Job: What Emerging Academic Leaders Should Do in the First Year. Establishing a robust foundation is essential for immediate success and long-term career development. The first year is critical for setting the tone of the leader's tenure, establishing effective leadership styles, and aligning with the organizational culture and mission. We have divided this chapter into four phases: preparation, launching, momentum, and consolidation. Each phase focuses on different aspects of transitioning, from letting go of past roles and building professional networks to managing personal and professional growth effectively.

Chapter 3: Leadership Styles and Levels. Effective leadership is not one-size-fits-all; it requires an understanding of different leadership styles and levels. In this chapter, we explore various leadership models, from transactional to transformational leadership, and discuss how different styles can be applied in academic settings. By gaining insight into their own leadership style and understanding the complexities of leadership levels within academic institutions, early-stage physicians can adapt their approach to different situations and effectively lead teams towards shared goals.

Chapter 4: Diversity, Equity, Inclusion, and Justice (DEIJ) in Academic Medicine. In this chapter, we highlight the persistent issues with racism and bias in academic medicine. We address the vital role of diverse faculty in improving medical education and patient care and examine the challenges of unconscious bias and its adverse effects on professional well-being, teamwork, patient care, recruitment, and retention. We offer suggestions for organizations and individuals on self-reflection, education, empathy, challenging stereotypes, seeking feedback, and continuous learning, to foster a healthcare system where belonging is a priority.

Chapter 5: Finances in Academic Medicine. In this chapter, we provide information that should prepare emerging physician leaders to make an informed decision about the challenging steps of joining an AMC with a competitive salary while contributing to patient-centered care, excellence in academics, and the financial health of the AMC.

Chapter 6: Conflict Management, Negotiations, and the Art of Hearing and Saying No in Academic Medicine. Conflict is an inevitable part of any dynamic organization, and academic institutions are no exception. In this chapter, we tackle the challenges of conflict management in academic environments and provide strategies for resolving conflicts constructively. By developing skills in communication, negotiation, and conflict resolution, early-stage physicians can navigate challenging situations with confidence and foster a culture of collaboration and mutual respect within their teams.

Chapter 7: Creating a Culture of Engagement and Combating Burnout. Managing physician well-being is multifaceted and requires a comprehensive strategy. In this chapter, we discuss how promoting a culture of engagement and addressing burnout preemptively can establish a supportive and enduring workplace. This enhances physicians' well-being, improves patient experience, and boosts organizational success. As physician leaders, it is crucial to cultivate an engaging atmosphere while being mindful of personal burnout and that of the team.

Chapter 8: Feedback in Academic Medicine. Feedback is a powerful tool for personal and professional growth, yet giving and receiving feedback effectively can be a daunting task. In this chapter, we explore the art of feedback in academic settings, discussing best practices for providing constructive feedback, receiving feedback with an open mind, and using feedback to drive continuous improvement. By mastering the art of feedback, early-stage physicians can create a culture of learning and development within their teams, driving innovation and excellence in academic medicine.

Chapter 9: Mentorship. Mentorship plays a pivotal role in the development of academic leaders, providing guidance, support, and inspiration along the way. In this chapter, we delve into the importance of mentorship in academic medicine and offer practical advice for finding and cultivating meaningful mentor–mentee relationships. By seeking out mentors who can offer valuable insights and perspectives, early-stage physicians can accelerate their growth as leaders and navigate the complexities of academic institutions with confidence and resilience.

Chapter 10: Academic Appointment and Promotions. In the final chapter of this book, we turn our focus to practical considerations for academic growth. From navigating promotion and tenure processes to building a strong professional network and balancing clinical and academic responsibilities, we offer actionable strategies for early-stage physicians to thrive in academic medicine. By mastering the practical aspects of academic growth, emerging leaders can position themselves for long-term success and make a lasting impact on the field of medicine.

In conclusion, *Emerging Leaders in Academic Medicine: A Concise Guide to Navigating the Path to Leadership* serves as a comprehensive roadmap for early-stage physicians seeking to cultivate their leadership potential in academic medicine. By exploring topics such as personal identity, leadership styles, conflict management, feedback, mentorship, and practical considerations for academic growth, this book equips readers with the knowledge and tools necessary to thrive as effective leaders in the complex landscape of academic institutions. Through self-reflection, skill development, and strategic planning, emerging leaders can navigate challenges, seize opportunities, and make a lasting impact on the future of healthcare and medical education.

Contents

About the Authors

Arjang Djamali, MD, MS, FASN, FACP was recently appointed the Maurice S. Segal, M.D., Chair of Medicine by the Tufts University Board of Trustees. Dr. Djamali joined Maine Medical Center (part of the MaineHealth system) in January 2022 as chair of medicine and director of the Adult Medicine Service Line. He now serves as Professor of medicine at TUSM and plays an important role in the clinical training of MD students who rotate in the MaineHealth system, including members of the Maine Track program. Prior to joining Maine Medical Center, Dr. Djamali was on the faculty of the University of Wisconsin-Madison (UW Health), where he rose through the ranks to the position of tenured professor of medicine and surgery and head of nephrology. As a transplant nephrologist and scientist with more than 200 manuscripts published in peer-reviewed journals, Dr. Djamali is considered a national leader in the areas of antibody-mediated processes and kidney transplant outcomes. He has been funded by the National Institutes of Health (NIH), foundations, and industry throughout his career and has been a member of the NIH's, Veterans Affairs Hospital's, and national societies' grant review panels; a member of advisory panels to the FDA and pharmaceutical industry; an invited speaker nationally and internationally; and a member of planning committees for national and international society meetings. Dr. Djamali has three INDs (investigational new drugs in clinical trials in transplants) and is the associate editor of Kidney360, the most recent publication from the American Society of Nephrology.

Fahad Aziz, MD, MBA, FASN is an Associate Professor of Medicine at the University of Wisconsin, where he serves as a faculty member in the Division of Nephrology. He specializes in providing comprehensive care for individuals with a wide range of kidney-related health issues, including those who have undergone kidney transplant. Dr. Aziz is dedicated to advancing the field through education and mentorship, as evidenced by his leadership of the Nephrology Fellowship Program at the university. As a transplant nephrologist, Dr. Aziz has published over 100 manuscripts in peer-reviewed journals and has authored and edited four books. In addition to his clinical and educational roles, he also serves as the Editor-in-Chief of the *Wisconsin Medical Journal*, highlighting his commitment to sharing medical knowledge and improving healthcare practices. Dr. Aziz has a strong passion for medical education and has a wealth of experience teaching nephrology to various learners, including medical and physician assistant students, internal medicine residents, and nephrology fellows. He also regularly conducts continuing medical education seminars for other healthcare professionals. His expertise is widely recognized, as he is an active member of the American College of Physicians, the American Society of Nephrology (ASN), and the American Society of Transplantation (AST). Dr. Aziz also contributes his insights and leadership as a board member of the National Kidney Foundation's Wisconsin Chapter, furthering his involvement in the medical community.

Dana Clark, MA is a highly accomplished professional with a rich academic background and extensive experience in academic affairs. She began her career in academia before transitioning into a career in academic medicine. Ms. Clark has contributed to the publication of 20 manuscripts and book chapters. Currently, Ms. Clark is Director of Faculty Appointments and Promotions at MaineHealth and is an Instructor at Tufts University School of Medicine. Always committed to knowledge sharing and working with others, Ms. Clark's current focus is on empowering junior faculty at the beginning of their careers and empowering them through academic pursuits and career advancement.

Chapter 1
Who Am I, and Who Do I Want to Be?

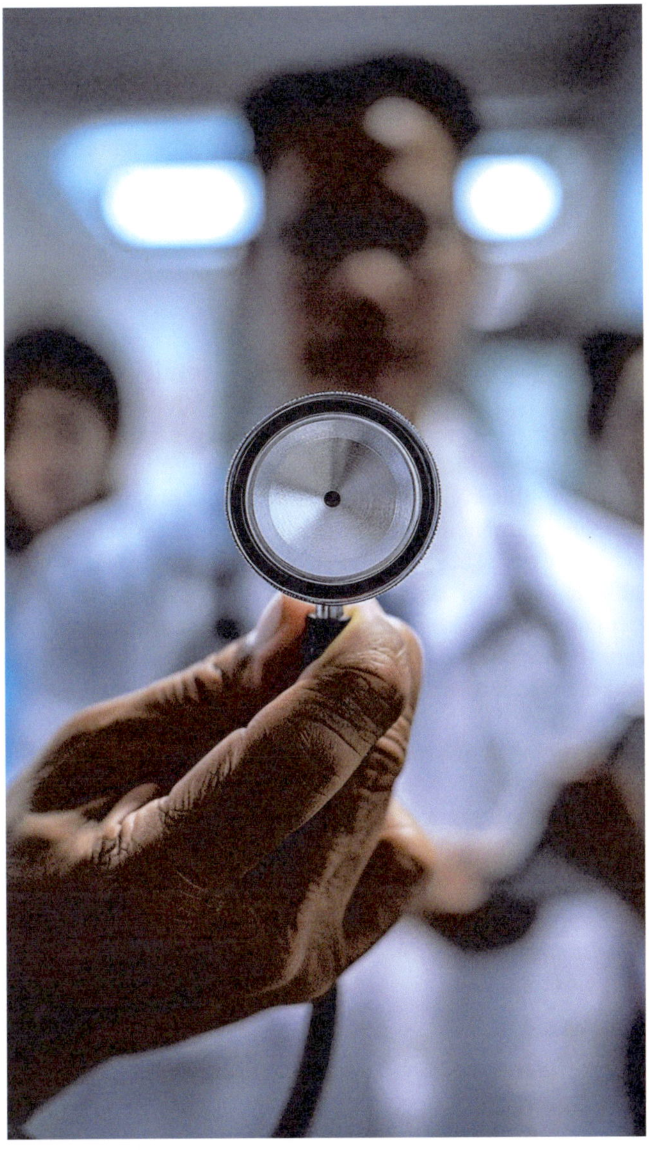

A. Djamali et al., *Emerging Leaders in Academic Medicine*,
https://doi.org/10.1007/978-3-031-80358-1_1

Case Presentation

Dr. Thompson is a young physician at an academic medical center, starting her first job after finishing her fellowship. Although she was known for her dedication to patient care and academic excellence while in training, Dr. Thompson feels overwhelmed when thinking about pursuing a leadership role and making a name for herself at her new institution. As a junior faculty, she has limited experience in administrative roles and feels uncertain about how to navigate the complexities of academic leadership. Moreover, balancing her clinical duties with research and teaching commitments leaves her with little time to develop her leadership skills. Dr. Thompson has a clear vision the strong leader she wants to become; however, the transition from who she was as a trainee to a leader her whole team supports and believes in seems daunting.

Introduction

While it may be too early to consider leadership positions as a trainee or junior faculty in an academic medical center, it is exactly the right time to think about where we want to see ourselves as leaders in the future and to plan for that future. Whether it is an academic medical center or private clinic setup, the leadership qualities presented in this book are essential to career progression and becoming a better physician and team member. "Leadership is much less about what you do and more about who you are." This powerful statement by Frances Hesselbein, founding President and Chairman of the Boards of Governors of the Leader-to-Leader Institution, explains how we as physician leaders must understand who we are and where we want to see ourselves in the future [1]. In this chapter, we will focus on defining a road map from where we are, and where we want to be.

Every journey starts with a road map (Fig. 1.1). For physician leaders, the journey to leadership begins with a roadmap or "mental map." This mental map helps us understand who we are and where we want to be; it helps us learn from our past, evaluate the present, and set a course to our desired future. Understanding and developing ourselves and influencing others through emotional intelligence are critical steps to their desired future.

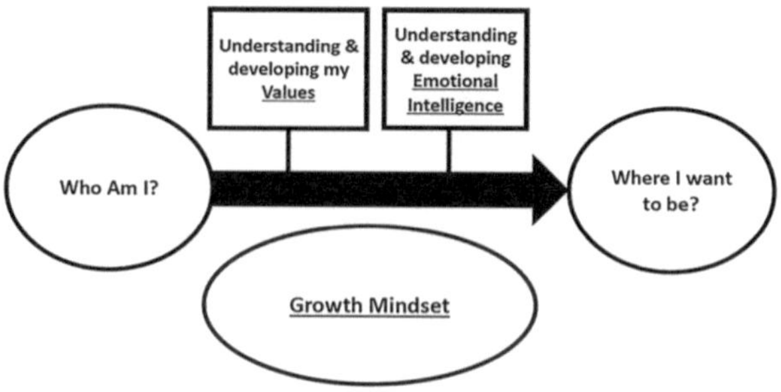

Fig. 1.1 Roadmap from "who am I" to "where I want to be"

Let's start with a simple example to understand the importance of a "mental map." Have you ever noticed an ant who is walking straight? If we place an obstacle in front of it, it will try to climb it, change its path to bypass the barrier, or go back and find another way. However, what the ant will not do is stop trying. That simple example explains an essential difference between people with a growth mindset and people with a fixed mindset. People with a growth mindset will never stop—no matter how big the obstacle is or how many times they try and fail—in their journey from "who I am" to "where I want to be." They see past experiences as lessons rather than a judgment and use them to build the future that they want.

Our personal belief systems and how those shape our mindsets are critical to developing a "mental map" for our journey to and through leadership roles. We are a product of many factors outside of our control—family, our communities, the training institutions we attended—in addition to our own individual personalities; no two people, even those who come from identical circumstances, will end up with the same belief systems or core values. Core values and personal belief systems act as a compass that guide our decisions and actions, and knowing your personal belief system allows you to set life goals that are achievable and deeply satisfying.

Understanding the impact of our belief system on life outcomes can be illuminated through the tale of two doctors, Dr. Adam and Dr. Brown, whose early careers were remarkably similar but whose later achievements diverged significantly. Both attended the same medical school and completed their residency in internal medicine at the same institution, setting them on seemingly parallel paths. Yet, as they approached retirement some 30–40 years later, their careers had taken very different directions. Dr. Adam concluded his career as the esteemed Dean of a medical school, leaving behind a legacy of substantial contributions to the field of medicine. He wrote five influential books, made significant contributions to several medical textbooks, and was published in over 200 peer-reviewed articles, securing his status as a key figure in the medical community with a lasting impact on medical science. In contrast, Dr. Brown retired as a respected general practitioner, an indispensable part of his local community who was valued for his compassion, empathy, and his commitment to remarkable patient care. Despite their differing journeys, both doctors exemplify the power of having a clear mental map where goals and personal values align—a vision for one's life and career. This clarity allowed each to navigate their unique paths successfully, demonstrating that success is not one dimensional but is instead defined by personal goals and sustained by a clear sense of purpose. Dr. Adam and Dr. Brown both reached the pinnacles of their respective careers by consistently aligning their actions with their long-term aspirations.

Who Am I and How Do People See Me?

For long-term success, the first and most crucial question to be answered is "Who am I?" Physician leaders in must answer this critical but challenging question. Successful physician leaders work hard to know themselves and to understand what motivates their behavior. After all, we are primarily judged based on our behavior, our actions, our spoken language, and our nonverbal communication (Fig. 1.2).

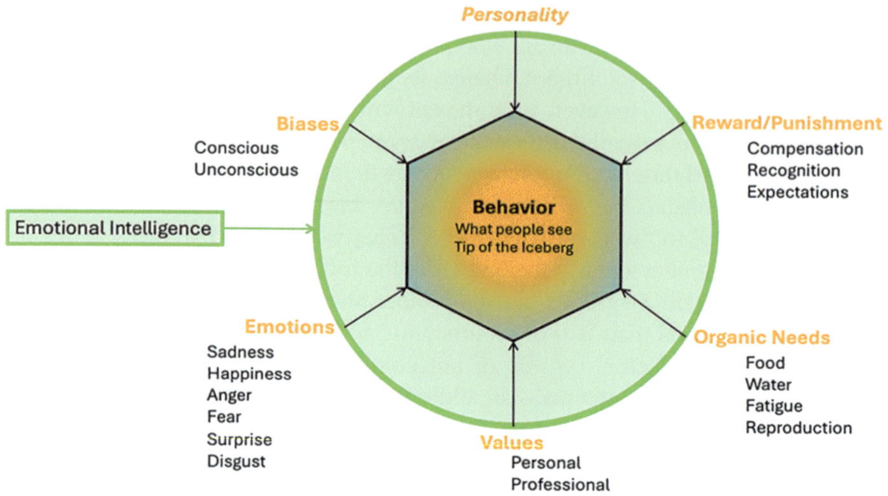

Fig. 1.2 Factors driving behavior and how to influence them

In this section, we will explain the "Tip of the Iceberg" model to help us understand our behaviors better (Fig. 1.2): The "Tip of the Iceberg" model is a metaphorical framework that illustrates how the visible actions of individuals, such as physician leaders, are just a small part of a larger range of underlying factors. This model suggests that the behaviors and decisions we witness are influenced by a complex interplay of internal and external elements, like how the visible part of an iceberg is supported by a larger hidden mass beneath the water's surface. It demonstrates how emotions, values, biases, personality, rewards and punishments, and organic needs all collectively shape behavior. A benefit of this model is that it highlights and helps us visualize the depth and complexity behind every action and interaction. Understanding this model can provide valuable insights into the motivations and drivers of behavior, which are essential for effective healthcare leadership and patient care.

Unveiling the Interplay: How Personality Shapes Our Behaviors

Learning effective leadership skills begins with a foundational step: self-knowledge. This entails our personality, response to reward and punishment, organic needs, our values, our emotions, and our conscious and unconscious biases. By gaining insight into these aspects, we not only chart a clear path toward our goals but also acquire the adaptability necessary to overcome challenges.

This self-awareness isn't an overnight achievement; rather, it's a gradual and intentional process. Delving into our strengths and acknowledging our weaknesses provides us with a roadmap for personal and professional growth. Moreover, recognizing, understanding, and accepting our personality is a cornerstone for developing emotional intelligence, which is a critical part of the leadership journey. As outlined by East Asian and Middle Eastern philosophy for millennia, the investment of time and intention into this ongoing process of self-discovery is pivotal. While it may be a lengthy endeavor, the dividends it pays in terms of becoming a more adept and resilient leader are immeasurable.

Of the six key variables affecting behavior, personality is the most powerful (Fig. 1.2). In general, our personality is determined by age seven, with small changes thereafter. Several tools allow personality profile evaluation, e.g., Myers-Briggs, Enneagram, and DiSC; we highly recommend that all resident trainees and early-stage physicians select at least one of these tests to determine their basic personality. Robert A. Rohm has extensively discussed the DiSC personality profiles in his book "Positive Personality Profiles" [2]. DiSC is a model that categorizes personalities according to four core traits based on whether we are outgoing or reserved, and whether we are task-oriented or people-oriented: dominance, influence, steadiness, and consciousness (Fig. 1.3). By comprehending these traits, we can gain insight

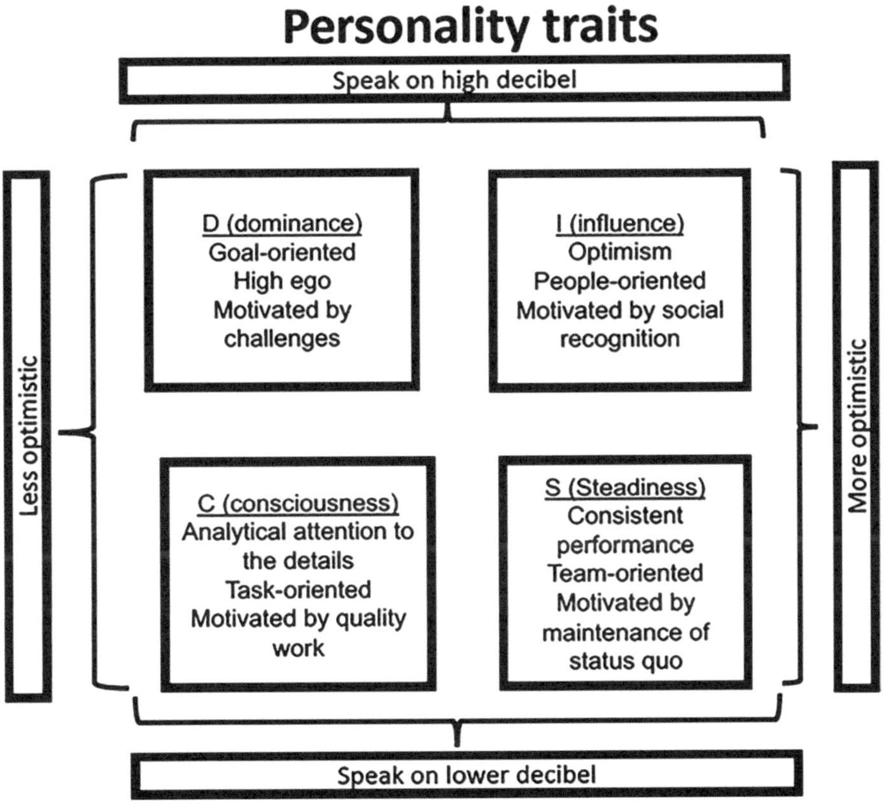

Fig. 1.3 Basic personality traits

into our own personality and communication styles, as well as those of the people around us. It is essential to recognize the advantages of each style, as well as the potential drawbacks. For example, your health system may ask your team to develop a new program and confirm there will be a financial reward associated with the successful completion of the project. Whereas a strong D's immediate response would be "What needs to be done? Let's get to work!" a strong I will ponder "Hmmm, I wonder who will be getting the bonus?" a strong S will think "Oh my, how exactly are we going to do this?" and finally a strong C will wonder "Why this change is needed? Isn't our current program good enough?" Each personality is naturally driven toward What (needing control); Who? (needing recognition); How? (needing appreciation); and Why? (needing quality answers).

In summary, a better understanding our own and our colleagues' personality profiles will help us improve communication with peers, bosses, and direct reports.

Behavioral Catalysts: Understanding the Effects of Rewards and Penalties

The dynamics of reward and punishment—such as compensation, recognition, and responsibilities—play a crucial role in influencing behavior across various facets of life, including work, personal development, and social interactions. Understanding the interplay of these factors is essential in comprehending how they shape our actions and decisions. Historically, the "carrot" (rewards) and "stick" (threats or punishments) have been mainstays of motivation (Fig. 1.2).

Let's consider a hospital network that introduces a performance-based bonus system. The goal is to improve patient experience and quality of care. Dr. Lee, who leads her medical team, is focused on improving communication skills and patient education. By enhancing active listening and ensuring that patients are well-informed about their conditions and treatments, Dr. Lee's team notices a significant increase in positive feedback from patients. Because of this achievement, the team is given a reward in the form of financial bonuses. This shows how financial incentives can motivate better performance and boost morale, creating a positive impact that benefits both healthcare providers and patients.

Conversely, punitive measures for noncompliance can also shape behavior. A local clinic introduces strict documentation standards for its EHR system, penalizing staff with salary deductions for failure to adhere to these requirements. Dr. Smith, who struggles with timely data entry, receives a salary deduction after repeated warnings, leading to frustration and a negative impact on his professional interactions. This example demonstrates how negative reinforcement can sometimes have unintended consequences, ultimately decreasing morale and performance instead of improving it. These are extreme examples, as one would hope that all physicians are self-driven to improve patient experience and professional compliance.

Recognition is another powerful motivator, as seen in the healthcare industry when Nurse Thompson receives the "Excellence in Nursing" award. This accolade not only honors her commitment and skills but also encourages her colleagues to elevate their standards of care. Similarly, Dr. Patel's feature in a medical society newsletter for his innovative work in rural healthcare inspires other physicians to undertake outreach initiatives, expanding the award's influence far beyond a single individual.

Expectations set within healthcare systems are also an important tool that can be used to drive behavior. Dr. Anderson, known for her dedication to patient-centered care, sets a high bar within her organization by aligning treatment plans with patients' individual health goals. Dr. Anderson clearly and regularly communicates these expectations to all of her team members, both faculty and trainees to create a formal culture within the team. Educational institutions, like medical schools, shape future healthcare practices by requiring students to engage in community service. This requirement, emphasized and explained by Dr. Anderson, fosters empathy and practical experience, equipping future professionals with the mindset to deliver compassionate, patient-focused care. Additionally, a hospital's goal to reduce hospital-acquired infections can lead to staff adopting stringent hygiene protocols, showcasing how clear objectives can enhance patient safety and care quality.

Through these examples, we can see how reward and punishment mechanisms, along with recognition and expectation setting, are fundamental to guiding behaviors. These principles not only affect individual actions but also have the potential to influence broader organizational culture and outcomes.

Foundational Beliefs: How Values Govern the Conduct of Physician Leaders

Personal and professional values are the fundamental beliefs and principles that shape how individuals and organizations act and make choices (Fig. 1.2). For physician leaders, professional values like integrity, respect, compassion, and excellence hold special significance as they directly influence the level of care given to patients and the working atmosphere they establish for their teams. It is important to note that personal values such as family, culture, religion, diet, exercise, and in general well-being are equally important drivers of behavior. Similarly, leaders should realize that personal and professional values may be generational and dynamic and change with time. For example, Baby Boomers, Generation X, Millennials, and Generation Z were raised in different social and political atmospheres and, therefore, correspond to different childhood upbringings and familial environments, which result in different values, wants, and needs in adulthood. A better understanding of characteristics that define each generation will help academic leaders to be more effective. We address few examples of professional values in the paragraphs below.

Integrity, for instance, motivates physician leaders to uphold the utmost ethical principles, guaranteeing that their behaviors align with professional and organizational codes of behavior. A physician leader with a strong value of integrity might be more vigilant in avoiding conflicts of interest, more diligent in maintaining patient confidentiality, and more committed to transparent communication. This creates a culture of trust, where patients feel secure in the care they receive, and team members feel confident in the leadership they follow.

Respect is an important value that influences how physician leaders interact with patients and colleagues. A leader who values respect will understand and appreciate the inherent worth of every person, regardless of their background or position. They will actively listen to their patients' concerns and preferences, involving them as partners in their own healthcare. Similarly, they will acknowledge the contributions of all team members, creating an inclusive environment where everyone feels valued and heard. For example, a physician leader who values respect may establish regular team meetings where all members, regardless of their rank, are encouraged to share their ideas and suggestions for enhancing patient care.

Compassion plays a crucial role in healthcare. It motivates physician leaders to show empathy and be responsive to the suffering of patients and the pressures their teams face. A leader who is compassionate not only offers emotional support to patients and their families but also cares about the well-being of their staff. They promote work-life balance and provide support to their team during tough times. For instance, during a challenging period like a flu epidemic, a compassionate physician leader may provide extra assistance to both patients and staff. They ensure that resources are available to handle the increased workload and emotional stress.

Excellence is a core principle that inspires physician leaders to constantly pursue the utmost quality in patient care and professional growth. Leaders who prioritize excellence will foster a culture of continuous learning, evidence-based practice, and innovation among their teams. They may, for instance, invest in advanced training for their staff, explore cutting-edge technologies that enhance patient outcomes, or spearhead research projects that advance medical knowledge.

In summary, the values upheld by physician leaders deeply impact their actions, decision-making, and the overall ethos of their healthcare organizations. By upholding values like integrity, respect, compassion, and excellence, physician leaders can ensure that they provide exemplary care to patients and foster a positive and productive work environment. Conversely, by respecting the dynamic and generational values of their team members, they can lead toward a shared vision of healthcare excellence.

Emotional Tides: The Impact of Positive and Negative Feelings on Physician Leadership

Emotions have a big impact on human behavior (Fig. 1.2). Emotions shape how we interact with other people, make decisions, and lead. Having highly positive emotions like happiness and empathy can improve a physician leader's ability to connect with patients and staff. It creates an atmosphere of trust and teamwork. For instance, a physician leader who feels empathetic toward a patient struggling with a chronic illness might go the extra mile to ensure that the patient receives comprehensive care and support, including coordinating with multidisciplinary teams to cover all aspects of the patient's well-being.

Conversely, negative emotions like frustration or anger can have detrimental effects on a physician leader's performance. Imagine a situation where a physician leader, after a week filled with stress from administrative tasks and challenging patient cases, starts to feel irritable and less communicative. Similarly, consider a colleague who recently lost a family member, loved one, or even a pet. Their situational sadness will undoubtedly impact their behavior, although you may not be privy to the reason behind this strong emotion. Emotional states can result in making cloudy judgments or having a dismissive attitude toward the concerns of team members, which can create a tense work environment and possibly compromise patient care. Such emotions can also result in decision fatigue, where the leader's decision-making quality declines over time due to emotional exhaustion.

Physician leaders may also find that their emotions can affect their ability to handle difficult situations and make fair decisions. A leader who feels anxious during a public health crisis might find it difficult to stay composed, which is essential for comforting the team and patients. This could lead to making rushed decisions without fully considering all possibilities, like hastily introducing new protocols that may not be well-planned or communicated effectively. For example, if the physician leader feels overwhelmed by the emotional toll of patient care, they could organize regular debriefing sessions for the team. This would provide an opportunity for everyone to express and address emotional challenges together. Not only does this help the leader manage their emotions, but it also supports the emotional well-being of the entire team. Ultimately, this leads to improved patient outcomes and a more positive work atmosphere. Later in the chapter, we will talk about the significance of cultivating emotional intelligence.

How can we control our emotions? What can we do so our emotions do not negatively impact our behavior? This is an incredibly challenging task, which requires a high level of emotional intelligence (Fig. 1.2). Emotional intelligence in a lifelong learning experience includes self-awareness, self-regulation, motivation, empathy, and social skills [3]. By recognizing and managing their emotions, leaders can stay calm under pressure, make better decisions, and create a supportive and collaborative team environment.

Organic Needs: The Influence of Our Biology on Our Behavior

As trivial as this may appear, organic or biological needs have been, and remain, a critical driver of animal and human behavior, leaders included (Fig. 1.2).

Basic Survival Needs

Our fundamental needs such as hunger, thirst, and sleep drive much of our behavior. For example, hunger can lead to behaviors aimed at finding and consuming food while the need for sleep influences our daily routines and productivity. A leader who understands their body's hunger or sleep schedule is better attune to when their best times are to schedule meetings, answer emails, or deal with demanding and delicate HR issues, for example.

Genetics

Our genetic makeup can predispose us to certain behaviors and traits, impacting our temperament, preferences, and even talents. A leader who understands their own inherent personality traits and recognizes those that their team members have can be more adaptable and accepting of the individuals on the team and how they act.

Hormones

Hormones are chemical messengers that regular various bodily functions and behaviors. How an individual's body produces and regulates cortisol, involved in the human stress response, can have great impact on how they behave during times of high workload and stress in the office. A leader can take into consideration employee's hormonal reactions by fostering an environment that supports well-being and recognizes the impact of hormones on mood and productivity.

Brain Structure and Function

Different regions of the brain are associated with specific behaviors. For example, the amygdala plays a key role in processing emotions like fear, while the prefrontal cortex is involved in decision-making and self-control. A good leader recognizes that each team member has unique manifestations of these cognitive processes and ways of processing information and reacting to external stimuli.

Evolutionary Influences

Many human behaviors have evolved to enhance our survival, group acceptance, and reproduction. Behaviors related to attachment and social bonding are critical of the cohesion of social groups and strong teams that can succeed in achieving common goals. A leader can take evolutionary influences into account by understanding how certain behaviors and tendencies have developed over time and how they manifest in the workplace.

Let's consider a few examples. Have you ever sent an email when hungry, that you regretted later? What about dozing-off during a presentation or meeting, assuming content and delivery were not boring? Or seeing a patient around noon time when hungry and thirsty? Or reading or hearing about risky sexual behavior in the work environment, where leaders put in peril family, career, and reputation? You get the point. Organic needs influence behavior and will therefore influence how we are seen, and how we see those around us.

In summary, people tolerate different levels of hunger, thirst, fatigue, sleep deprivation, etc. None of these organic needs are excuses for inappropriate behavior; rather, understanding human needs allows us to better understand ourselves and how these needs manifest in each of us. Good leaders make sure they do not allow organic needs and biology impinge on their leadership to ensure they show up each day as they care for patients or attend important meetings with their team, peers, or boss.

Unseen Influences: The Effect of Biases on Physician Leadership Behavior

Our individual beliefs and preferences, whether conscious or unconscious, can impact our behaviors and decision-making processes (Fig. 1.2). These effects extend to all aspects of patient care and team management. For example, a physician leader may unknowingly associate certain health behaviors with specific demographics, leading to a different approach in patient treatment plans. As a result, there may be variations in the quality of care, with some patients receiving a higher standard of treatment than others due to the physician's inherent biases. When it comes to decision-making, these biases can result in either over-treatment or under-treatment of conditions, as leaders may interpret symptoms or patient testimonies based on their biases. This has the potential to influence patient outcomes.

Addressing diversity, equity, and inclusion is a key component of modern leadership skills and is one we address more fully in Chap. 4 of this book. When it comes to leading a team, bias can also affect decisions regarding mentorship, promotion, and recruitment. Let's imagine a situation where a physician leader unconsciously favors colleagues of the same gender over equally competent colleagues of other genders due to an unconscious bias. As a result, colleagues of their own gender consistently receive more leadership opportunities and support compared to their counterparts of other genders. This unintentionally creates a work environment that marginalizes team members and hampers growth within the organization. Such biases not only impact team dynamics and morale but also limit the diversity of perspectives needed for innovative approaches and comprehensive patient care.

The consequences of biases held by physician leaders contribute to inequalities in healthcare systems. For example, let's consider a situation where a physician leader unknowingly has a bias against older patients, assuming they are less likely to benefit from aggressive treatments. Consequently, this leader may suggest less advanced treatment options for older patients compared to younger individuals with similar health conditions. This bias based on age can result in unequal healthcare outcomes and perpetuate disparities in healthcare related to age.

To address these biases, it is important for physician leaders to regularly reflect on their own actions, participate in bias training, and establish fair protocols for patient care and personnel decisions. Creating a culture that values diversity and promotes equal treatment is crucial. Most institutions now offer regular unconscious bias trainings, and these courses can provide concrete methods and plans to help us reduce our own unconscious biases. By actively taking steps and continuing to learn, physician leaders can contribute to eliminating biases that affect their behavior and the healthcare system. This will result in providing fair and effective care to all patients and fostering a more inclusive workplace.

Summary of Iceberg Model

The Iceberg model is a helpful metaphor that allows us to comprehend both the observable and hidden aspects of human behavior. Like an iceberg, the majority of what influences our actions is concealed beneath the surface. This model suggests that behaviors are shaped by a combination of internal factors, including our emotions, our values (which guide our ethical choices), our biases (both known and unknown, subtly influencing our judgments), our personality traits (dictating our consistent patterns of behavior), the rewards or punishments we anticipate (motivating our actions), and our fundamental organic needs (such as hunger and thirst). Together, these factors make up the bulk of the iceberg below the waterline, supporting and shaping the visible behaviors that appear above the surface. Understanding this model is essential for those in leadership positions, such as physician leaders, as it emphasizes the significance of self-awareness and the impact of one's internal world on external leadership and decision-making.

Emotional Intelligence

The concept of emotional intelligence (the "green circle" in Fig. 1.2) was first introduced by John Mayer and Peter Salovey in 1990, defining it as the ability to understand and manage one's own emotions as well as recognize and influence the emotions of others. The idea gained widespread recognition in 1995 when psychologist Daniel Goleman published his seminal book "Emotional Intelligence" in which he argued that emotional intelligence is a crucial factor in effective leadership and often more important than traditional measures of intelligence such as IQ and technical skills. Emotional Intelligence is critical to our journey from who we are to where we want to be and is a key component in human behavior and acts as a navigational tool for physician leaders to understand and influence the behaviors at the surface—the "tip of the iceberg" in the Iceberg model. It emphasizes the need to be cognizant of our emotions and the emotions of those around us. For physician leaders, developing emotional intelligence is crucial for effectively managing the myriad factors that influence our actions and leadership style. This involves examining the emotional factors that influence decision-making and communication, enabling individuals to respond in a way that acknowledges the intricacies of their team's and patients' emotional well-being. The utilization of emotional intelligence can result in professional interactions that are not only efficient but also compassionate and empathetic.

Most physicians, especially in academic medical centers, are not traditionally trained in teamwork, which is vital for success in healthcare. The high-stakes world of medicine demands collaboration for more cohesive interprofessional teams, better patient outcomes, and individual growth. In the medical field, where the focus is often on direct care and efficiency, the value of emotional intelligence can sometimes be overlooked.

To emerge as effective team players, physicians must harness emotional intelligence to forge strong interpersonal relationships and manage team dynamics. As such, emotional intelligence is not just a beneficial attribute but a necessary one for physicians who aim to lead with empathy and efficiency in the ever-evolving landscape of healthcare. This skill set is not innate to many in the field and often requires deliberate effort and learning to master. Thankfully, emotional intelligence is a skill that can be learned and developed.

Emotional intelligence as a principle of leadership has evolved significantly in the past few decades. Goleman identified five key components of Emotional Intelligence: self-awareness, self-regulation, motivation, empathy, and social skills. These five components fall into two broad categories—managing ourselves (self-awareness, self-regulation, motivation) and managing others (empathy, social skills).

Managing Ourselves

Learning self-awareness, self-regulation, and motivation to better manage ourselves is important as these skills enhance our ability to navigate complex situations, build stronger relationships, and achieve our goals. Understanding our own emotions, strengths, weaknesses, and values allows us to make better decisions and aligns actions with goals by recognizing how our emotions affect our behavior and how we are perceived by others. Managing our emotions and impulses, staying calm under pressure, and maintaining control over actions help us respond thoughtfully rather than reactively in situations, reducing stress during difficult times and improving our ability to handle challenges.

Self-Awareness

Self-awareness stands as a pivotal skill, enabling us to grasp the nuances of our moods, emotions, and drives, along with their profound impact on those around us. This cognitive ability is not merely a commendable trait but a cornerstone for realizing our utmost personal potential and enhancing our overall effectiveness. However, delving into self-awareness goes beyond a surface-level understanding of our strengths and positive attributes—it involves a comprehensive exploration of our weaknesses and the shadows within us, completing the intricate equation of self-awareness. In acknowledging our strengths, we illuminate the positive facets of our identity, but true self-awareness requires an honest confrontation with our vulnerabilities and the less favorable aspects of our character. This comprehensive self-examination lays the groundwork for a more authentic and profound understanding of ourselves.

The challenge lies in the inherent human tendency to perceive ourselves through a subjective lens, often veering toward an idealized version of who we are. Paradoxically, our capacity for objective self-reflection is hindered, making it difficult to perceive ourselves as others do. This asymmetry in perception becomes more pronounced when juxtaposed with our ability to readily form assessments of others based on our limited interactions with them.

Interestingly, individuals who radiate authenticity tend to be more self-aware. They navigate the delicate balance between recognizing their strengths and vulnerabilities, embracing both the light and the shadows within. Authenticity, in essence, becomes a beacon guiding us toward a more profound understanding of ourselves, enabling us to bridge the gap between self-perception and how others perceive us. In the intricate dance of self-awareness, the willingness to explore the entirety of our being, both the luminous and the obscure, propels us toward a more holistic and genuine connection with ourselves and the world around us.

Self-Regulation

At the core of personal and professional efficacy lies the art of self-regulation—an indispensable skill that empowers us to navigate the intricate landscape of our emotions and behavior. Mastering the ability to lead oneself is an endeavor of profound significance, constituting the fundamental challenge before assuming the responsibility of leading others. Indeed, self-leadership serves as the crucible for developing the qualities necessary to guide and inspire those around us.

Self-regulation, in essence, is the compass that guides our actions, allowing us to respond thoughtfully to the myriad challenges and emotions encountered in both personal and professional spheres. It transcends the mere management of emotions; it encapsulates the wisdom to steer our behavior in alignment with our goals and values. By conquering the formidable task of self-leadership, we lay the groundwork for authentic and impactful leadership of others.

Moreover, self-regulation serves as a cornerstone for personal growth and professional development. It entails a conscious effort to understand the triggers and patterns governing our responses, enabling us to make informed choices that align with our overarching objectives. This self-awareness, coupled with the ability to regulate our behavior judiciously, establishes a fertile ground for sustained success.

Self-regulation is based on the following essential behaviors:

- **Openness and Transparency**: Transparency is about being open to others and their ideas without secret agendas. There should always be a policy of openness, where we should be able to hear from all the people around us. We all have blind spots in our life, and openness helps us to visualize these blind spots from others' eyes. This ultimately allows us to learn and progress. If we are approachable, people will walk into our daily lives and help us achieve our higher goals. Transparency creates trust, and trust leads to making meaningful connections.
- **Willingness**: Self-aware leaders know their weaknesses and self-regulate with their willingness to change. They are open to positive and negative feedback without getting defensive, which helps them grow continually.
- **Understanding Our Values**: As mentioned above, defining and understanding one's values are paramount. True leaders self-regulate themselves based on the values they believe in. As a famous saying goes, "It's the character that anchors us well."
- **Consistency**: Most of us strive to have some level of stability in life. Consistency in daily life brings a certain degree of predictability, which we all crave. Self-awareness helps us integrate consistency into our behaviors, actions, and approach. The first thing which needs to be consistent is our behavior and attitude. Imagine working with a coworker or a boss whose behavior and attitude are inconsistent. One day they may be pleasant and all smiles; the next, they are frustrated, annoyed, and angry.

While the medical field can be stressful, we must control our emotions to positively influence the people working with us. We must show up daily in the same way regardless of what's happening. This creates a strong feeling of security among the people working around us. Our team members should know they can count on us during the most stressful times.

Over time I understood the importance of consistent behavior and its effect on the people working around me. As leaders in academic medicine, sometimes we undervalue how much our attitude, behavior, and comments affect others, and this impact is real. Let me give a personal example here. In our transplant clinic, we perform transplant kidney biopsies every day. My day for doing kidney biopsies is every Monday. As I start my day earlier, I want to start my procedures. The nurses working on Monday are so used to my consistent behavior that they begin getting patients ready for their biopsy as soon as possible and call ultrasound to help us with the biopsies on the early side, as they know I would be available earlier and would like to finish the procedures sooner. I was often told that the nurses appreciated my consistency on biopsy day, making it more predictable for them.

Let me be clear on one more thing: consistency is not about never changing. We must know that, as dynamic leaders, change is inevitable and necessary. Consistency is all about how we deal with that change, and our approach to that change should be consistent, giving our team a sense of dependability. Without consistency, we cannot create a culture of trust and reliability.

Motivation

Motivation is exceptionally critical for leading others. Learning what drives our actions, whether internal satisfaction or external validation, helps us stay focused and resilient. Motivation fuels our persistence and enthusiasm and enables us to overcome obstacles as they come up to keep us focused on long-term objectives. Motivated physician leaders have the drive to get things done. Their passion is contagious. They enjoy new challenges and stay optimistic even during the most challenging times. The team can always look at them to keep going. Lack of energy and motivation is the enemy of leadership. A lack of inspiration in physician leaders creates a leadership deficit.

Managing Others

Increasing our empathy and growing our social skills to better manage others is important as it allows for better communication, conflict resolution, and influence within and over a team. Being in tune with the emotional needs of team members and being able to communicate that understanding allow leaders to create a more emotionally intelligent team. This, in turn, can create a more positive and productive work environment.

Empathy

Empathy is the ability to understand the emotional makeup of other people, both sensing others' emotions and imagining how others might be thinking or feeling. Physician leaders increase their influence on the people around them through empathy. What we say is important, but how others feel around us is even more critical. With strong empathy, physician leaders direct the people to their vision and ultimately to the desired direction. They understand the power of effective communication and can connect with others on a deeper level.

Types of Empathy

1. Affective empathy refers to the ability to understand others' emotions and feelings. Understanding the emotions of those on our team plays a vital role in fostering emotional connections and creating a supportive environment. This is done by the building of trust that results in sharing feelings, enhances communication, reduces conflict, and fosters inclusivity.
2. Cognitive empathy, also sometimes referred to as perspective-taking, refers to the ability to understand the perspective of others without necessarily sharing their emotional experience. Authentic cognitive empathy is an important tool for leaders as it allows them to demonstrate they understand something a team member is dealing with even when it is something the leader has never themselves experienced. Benefits of cognitive empathy also include improved communication, increased inclusivity, and stronger team relationships.

Ways to Show Empathy

Physicians should take the following steps to show their empathy for other people:

1. *Radical listening to others*: Radical listening allows us to fully understand and respond to another person's needs and emotions. It allows us to balance our emotional understanding with logical analysis of a situation, in turn helping us offer effective and supportive solutions. Radical listening helps us process and organize information more clearly, which allows for reduced misunderstandings.
2. *Ask open-ended questions to understand better*: Open-ended questions build trust between people by encouraging sharing thoughts and feelings. It promotes a deeper exploration of feelings and ideas, reducing assumptions on both sides of the conversation.
3. *Recall similar experiences of our own*: When appropriate, sharing similar experiences can enhance the empathetic connection between leader and team member and provides support to someone facing a problem. Validating feelings and providing perspective strengthens connections and encourages openness within teams.
4. *Paraphrasing*: Paraphrasing enhances understanding, validation, and connection as it clarifies communication and builds trust. By paraphrasing, we can confirm that we have accurately understand the other person's message, reducing or

removing assumptions and ensuring all parties are on the same page regarding the topic under discussion.
5. *Mirroring*: Mirroring allows us to establish a rapport and communicate that we are on the same page as the person we are talking to. By mirroring someone's body language, tone of voice, or expressions, it signals that we are attuned to the emotions and experiences they are sharing.
6. *Supportive body language*: Supportive body language reinforces the verbal communication that is taking place. This helps re-emphasize the cues that encourage openness and create an emotional connection.

Benefits of Empathy

1. *Empathy results in social well-being, leading to psychological and physiological well-being*: empathy strengthens relationships and promotes prosocial behavior, leading to reduced conflict. It also enhances emotional regulation, which in turn has been shown to increase work-life satisfaction and reduces stress and anxiety. These social and psychological benefits themselves impact physiological well-being, lowering blood pressure, boosting immune function, and promoting longevity.
2. *Empathy leads to emotional regulation*: The self-awareness and perspective-taking required for empathy also promote enhanced coping strategies and improved interpersonal skills. These are key to understanding and managing our own emotions more effectively.
3. *Empathy helps overcome emotional numbness and creates a sense of connection with life*: Empathy allows us to connect with our emotions and the meaningful connections created when empathy is engaged helps fight the emotional numbness that can lead to a deeper sense of isolation. These interpersonal connections can build stronger relationships and engagement with the world around us.
4. *Empathy helps to build teams*: Empathy improves communication, builds trust, enhances collaboration, reduces conflict, and encourages engagement and inclusivity. It is the glue that holds effective teams together, fostering a positive and productive work environment.

Social Skills

Physician leaders with strong social skills are influential in leading the charge expertly and building and leading teams. Social skills allow individuals to navigate various social situations with ease, whether it be in a professional setting or in personal relationships. Furthermore, social skills are essential for networking and building connections. People with strong social skills can establish rapport with others, making it easier to form meaningful relationships. They can effortlessly engage in conversations, actively listen, and show genuine interest in others. This ability to connect with people enables them to expand their network, create opportunities, and collaborate effectively.

In addition, social skills are crucial for leadership. Leaders with strong social skills can inspire and motivate others. They understand the importance of building trust and fostering a positive work environment. By demonstrating empathy and understanding, they can effectively address the needs and concerns of their team members, leading to increased productivity and overall success.

Overall, social skills are not just about being friendly but rather about using that friendliness to connect with others, understand their perspectives, and work toward a common goal. They are essential for effective communication, networking, and leadership. Developing and honing these skills can greatly enhance one's ability to navigate social interactions and achieve success in various aspects of life.

Exploring Mindsets: The Power of Fixed Versus Growth Perspectives

Embracing a growth mindset is indispensable for physician leaders who are committed to continuous development. In the intricate realm of healthcare, fostering a culture of growth mindset becomes not just advantageous but essential. For young physicians, understanding the art of cultivating this mindset is a crucial aspect of their professional journey. Instilling and nurturing a growth mindset is not merely an individual endeavor but a collective commitment to the perpetual evolution of medical knowledge and practice. By internalizing this approach, physician leaders pave the way for a resilient and adaptive healthcare system that thrives on continuous learning and improvement.

The significance of a growth mindset was imparted to me early in my career by seasoned mentors during my residency. Their sage advice echoes through time: never turn down the opportunity to perform a procedure, regardless of its perceived insignificance. This philosophy underscores a fundamental principle—every procedure, regardless of scale, offers a unique learning experience. Physician growth, it was emphasized, hinges on navigating the professional journey with an open mind, a readiness to absorb knowledge at any given moment. The wisdom lies in recognizing that each learning opportunity, no matter how minor, contributes to the expansive landscape of medical expertise. This mindset not only propels personal development but also serves as a cornerstone for the advancement of healthcare in general.

Growth Mindset

The two key factors in cultivating a growth mindset are core values and emotional intelligence.

1. **Understanding and Developing Core Values**: Our core values are the bedrock of our leadership, and they shape our actions. Without strong core values, leaders lack trustworthiness and transparency in their intentions. A lack of values has an impact on both the leader and those around them. Before we can become influential leaders, it is essential to comprehend our core values, and we must pledge to abide by them. We believe in these core values for any leader:

    - **Integrity**: Integrity is doing the right thing regardless of the outcome, even when no one is watching. As John Maxwell said, "Integrity is important in building relationships and is the foundation upon which many other qualities for success are built, such as respect, dignity, and trust" [4]. Leaders who demonstrate integrity gain trust among their colleagues, are not afraid of the truth, and know how to stand up for their beliefs. Integrity is a leader's best friend.
    - **Honesty**: Being an honest leader means you do not deceive others by giving out misleading information. Honesty is essential for any leader because it allows them to build trust, apologize when necessary, and show vulnerability. Honesty is more than just not lying; it's the commitment to know they understand the truth and then lead with it.
    - **Discipline**: Self-discipline is crucial for the development of leaders. It is the essential characteristic that separates those who achieve success from those who don't. The three most vital C's of self-discipline are consistency, communication, and common sense. Consistency in values, behaviors, and moods is critical for leaders. People with inconsistent moods, behaviors, and values cannot attain the confidence of those around them.
    - **Respect**: Leaders are always respectful of the people around them. To earn respect, it's essential to give respect. Leaders listen to the people around them, regardless of their thoughts and approaches. Listening is the basis of respecting others. Valuing others' opinions is also an important way of showing respect. Leaders say thank you often and apologize quickly.
    - **Accountability**: High levels of accountability among leaders build trust within teams. Knowing that their leader will take responsibility for their decisions increases team members' confidence in the leader. Accountability helps leaders to be humble and welcome the assistance of others.
    - **Humility**: Humility is crucial to developing a growth mindset. It helps physicians to learn from anyone. In his interview with Oprah in April of 2001, Nelson Mandela said, "Humility is the most important thing you should have to succeed. If you make people realize you are no threat to them, they will take no time to embrace you" [5]. These powerful statements define genuine humility and why it's crucial for leaders. It is also essential to understand that humility does not equal weakness or being soft; it gives young leaders freedom from arrogance and strengthens them. Without humility, it's not possible to achieve a growth mindset.

2. **Incorporating Emotional Intelligence into Growth Mindset**: incorporating emotional intelligence into growth mindset creates a robust framework for continuous personal and professional development. It enhances our learning abilities, increases resilience, builds stronger relationships, and increases our self-awareness.

Conclusion

Successful physician leaders embark on their career path with a crucial self-inquiry: Who am I? This reflection is the starting point for understanding their own strengths, weaknesses, and ambitions. As they define their personal and professional vision, they adopt a growth mindset, which allows them to view challenges as opportunities for development rather than obstacles. They recognize that their advancement is rooted in core values and emotional intelligence, essential qualities that guide their interactions and decision-making.

Armed with a clear and detailed plan for reaching their goals, these leaders not only work on their own growth but also invest in the development of their colleagues. They understand the importance of cultivating a supportive environment where everyone is encouraged to learn and improve. By fostering this culture of continuous growth and self-improvement, they not only achieve their own vision but also inspire and elevate those around them, creating a collective drive toward excellence in their field.

Take-Home Points

- Understanding and developing growth mindset is essential for physician leaders to succeed in their career.
- Successful physician leaders understand the roadmap of where they are and where they want to be.
- Successful physician leaders recognize the significance of cultivating emotional intelligence, or the green circle, both for comprehending themselves and those around them.

References

1. Collins J. Hesselbein on leadership. 2022. https://www.jimcollins.com/article_topics/articles/hesselbein.html#:~:text=Early%20in%20this%20book%2C%20Frances,more%20about%20who%20you%20are. Accessed 3 Dec 2023.
2. Rohm RA. Positive personality profiles. 3rd ed. Personality Insights Press; 2018.
3. Goleman D. Emotional intelligence: why it can matter more than IQ. Bloomsbury Publishing; 2015.
4. Maxwell JC. Top 500 John C. Maxwell quotes (2024 update). 2024. https://quotefancy.com/john-c-maxwell-quotes. Accessed 4 Dec 2023.
5. Afreaka. Nelson Mandela on Oprah Winfrey. 2001/2013.

Chapter 2
Starting Your New Job: What Emerging Academic Leaders Should Do in the First Year

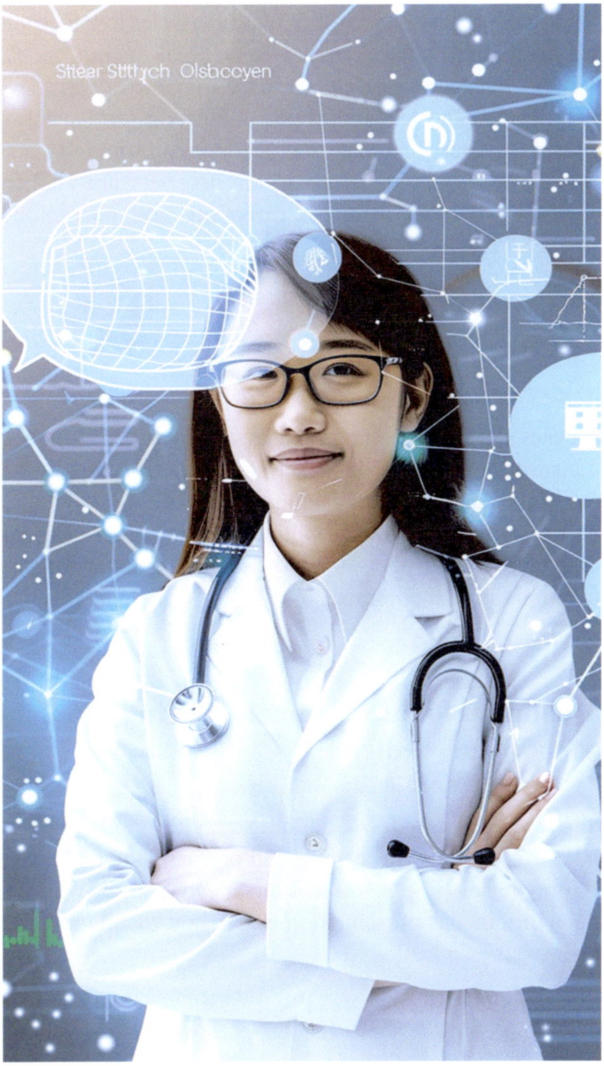

A. Djamali et al., *Emerging Leaders in Academic Medicine*,
https://doi.org/10.1007/978-3-031-80358-1_2

Case Presentation

Dr. Chen recently completed her fellowship program and is starting her first academic job as an assistant professor at a university hospital different to where she trained. This is a significant achievement for a young doctor; however, it also presents substantial challenges, particularly in the first year as an academic medical physician leader. Dr. Chen must focus on her clinical work while establishing herself in teaching, research, and scholarship to achieve long-term success.

Transitioning to a new clinical setup, culture, colleagues, and supervisors can be stressful. This significant milestone in life can bring challenges such as self-doubt and the pressure associated with an academic medical institution. The first year in roles like Dr. Chen's is crucial, setting the tone for her time at the institution and establishing her priorities and leadership style. For long-term success in her career, Dr. Chen needs to introduce herself to the academic community and align herself with the university's mission. Her efforts in the first year are vital for building her reputation, influencing her department's direction, and positioning herself as a forward-thinking leader in her field.

Introduction

This chapter focuses on new physician leaders as they begin their careers at academic medical institutions. It provides essential advice for their first academic year, emphasizing the importance of establishing solid professional connections, understanding the institutional culture, and defining their professional goals. By concentrating on these fundamental aspects, leaders can pave the way for sustained success in their academic and clinical pursuits.

First-Year Roadmap to Success for Emerging Physician Leaders in Academic Medicine

To succeed in the short and long term, building a solid foundation in the first year as a physician leader is essential. We recommend breaking the first year in a new leadership role into four phases (Fig. 2.1). Looking ahead to know where you are headed but maintaining focus in the present moment is key to intentionality and setting goals when starting out as a leader.

- Phase 1: Preparation phase
- Phase 2: Launching phase
- Phase 3: Momentum phase
- Phase 4: Consolidation phase

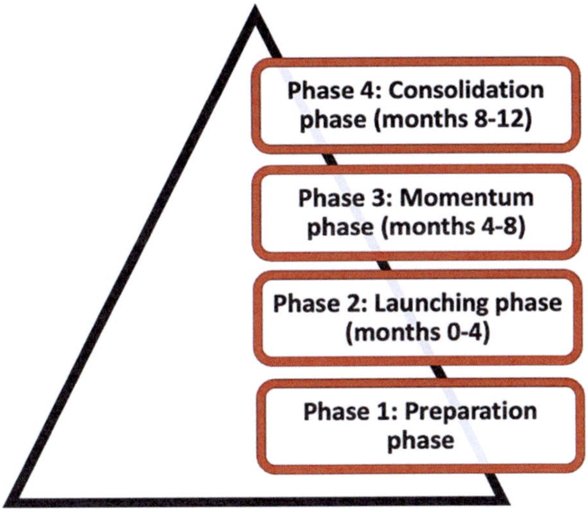

Fig. 2.1 First-year roadmap

Phase 1: Preparation Phase: Laying the Foundation (Before the Start of the Job)

The preparation phase can help us set ourselves up for success. When all the elements come together, it allows us to understand the organizational landscape to better inform decisions; it lets us establish initial connections with key stakeholders and team members to begin gaining support and building trust from the start; and it allows us to better define clear, achievable goals in our personal roadmap.

1. **Shifting Focus from Previous Role**: Transitioning from a trainee physician to an attending physician is a significant achievement in a physician's career journey. While the security of supervision during training is comforting, attending physicians, especially leaders, need to step out of their comfort zone to advance to the next level of decision-making. To quote the renowned author and attorney Roy T. Bennett, "You never change your life until you step out of your comfort zone; change begins at the end of your comfort zone" [1].

   Trainee physicians frequently form deep emotional bonds with their training institutions, and transitioning away from these ties can be difficult; however, it is crucial to do as they assume new roles at various institutions with more significant challenges. Releasing past emotional attachments enables physician leaders to embrace their new duties and chances for growth wholeheartedly.
2. **Configure the Energy Management System**: Navigating the first year in an academic medical center as a young physician leader can be intense and challenging as it is fulfilling and transformative. Effective energy management is critical, focusing on caring for the mind, maintaining physical health, and building a supportive network. Embracing a calm and focused mindset and a stable personal life sets the stage for success in this demanding setting.

A physician leader needs a support system to help them transition into their new role. Colleagues, mentors, and family members provide valuable emotional and professional assistance. As Michael Watkins, a renowned writer, highlights in his book The First 90 Days, effective leadership involves leveraging the support and influence of others in the organization [2]. This inclusive strategy enhances personal resilience and enables young physicians to inspire and lead within their medical institutions.

3. **Recognizing the Value of Family Stability**: Renowned Canadian and American activist and retired actor Michael J. Fox once wisely remarked, "Family is not an important thing. It's everything" [3]. Prioritizing family is crucial, particularly for physician leaders navigating transitions. A robust support system at home is vital as they embrace new responsibilities. Attending to family requirements and securing their backing can significantly impact a physician's professional achievements. This equilibrium empowers leaders to focus on their roles with the assurance that their personal lives are stable. Moreover, valuing family can lead to increased personal fulfillment, ultimately enhancing leadership and motivational skills in the workplace [2].
4. **Understanding Time Pressure**: As a new physician leader, managing time efficiently can be challenging. While in training, young physicians likely had to supervise attendings to help with scheduling and duties. As an independent physician leader, handling time effectively to balance patient care, administrative tasks, and personal growth is crucial. Famous leadership teacher Stephen R. Covey advised, "The key is not to prioritize what's on your schedule, but to schedule your priorities" [4]. Developing strong time management skills early on will help physician leaders navigate challenges and fulfill professional responsibilities without feeling overwhelmed. Robin Sharma emphasized, "Time management is life management" [5]. Physician leaders need to comprehend this and prepare early to improve their time management skills before starting the job.
5. **Navigating the Learning Curve**: Transitioning to independent physician leaders can be challenging for new physicians. Although medical training provides a solid base, applying that knowledge in real-life scenarios can be daunting. To adapt to new protocols, technologies, and patient demographics, physician leaders must keep learning and growing professionally. Attending workshops, engaging in CME programs, and seeking input from peers and mentors can all aid in bridging the theory-to-practice gap.
6. **Developing New Teams and Networks**: Establishing strong relationships and forming a team is critical for a successful transition. Working closely with colleagues, nurses, and other healthcare professionals is vital in academic medicine. For new physician leaders, investing time in networking within their institution and the medical community is crucial. Before commencing their roles, physician leaders should focus on understanding their team and identifying key allies. Patrick Lencioni famously said, "Teamwork starts with trust. To build trust, we must let go of our need to be invulnerable" [6]. This strategy fosters a cooperative and encouraging atmosphere, setting the stage for effective leadership.

7. **Striking the Right Balance in Pace**: Leaders must find a balance when navigating transitions. Moving too quickly can lead to errors and burnout, while moving too slowly may cause missed chances and a lack of progress. Joyce Meyer once said, "Patience is not simply the ability to wait—it's how we behave while we're waiting" [7]. Setting achievable goals and timelines is critical to steady progress while ensuring quality care and professional growth. Regularly reviewing the progress and making necessary changes will help maintain a sustainable and effective pace [8]. Considering and practicing finding the perfect pace before beginning the job is essential.
8. **Grasping Institutional Culture**: This is probably one of the most important pieces of leadership, regardless of which stage you belong to. Every academic institution has its unique culture, shaped by its history, values, and norms. Even before starting their jobs, physician leaders must try to deeply understand this culture, exploring surface-level aspects and underlying principles. Embracing the institution's mission is crucial as it lays the groundwork for its purpose and overall goals. Leaders can steer their actions and decisions in the right direction by aligning with these core values and aspirations. Understanding the organizational structure, including roles, responsibilities, and hierarchy, is also crucial. This knowledge helps navigate bureaucratic processes, avoiding obstacles and improving workflow efficiency. By grasping the culture, mission, strategic priorities, and organizational structure, physician leaders acquire respect, and the knowledge and skills needed to navigate the intricacies of academia, focusing their efforts on success in this constantly evolving environment. It's essential to carefully observe and understand the institutional culture before beginning a new job for a successful start.
9. **Identifying Mentors**: Finding the perfect mentor is essential for young physician leaders in medical institutions. Mentors provide more than just career advice; they offer support, guidance, and invaluable wisdom to help navigate the complexities and opportunities of academic medicine. Physician leaders must begin searching for suitable mentors before entering the new role. As Oprah Winfrey wisely states, "A mentor is someone who allows you to see the hope inside yourself" [9]. Therefore, physician leaders should actively seek mentorship opportunities, remain open to different perspectives, and welcome the opportunity to grow and succeed in their careers.
10. **Considering Leadership Purpose**: As a physician leader, it is crucial to regularly reflect on one's leadership purpose and align the challenges faced with progress and aspirations. Start by understanding why this role exists and identifying the most meaningful aspects. This self-reflection helps maintain a connection to the core reasons behind the professional journey. By clarifying motivations, responsibilities can be navigated with a clear sense of direction and purpose.

    Writing down specific objectives and questions enhances clarity of purpose as a leader. Consider whether and how the position aligns with personal career aspirations and how current duties contribute to professional growth. Assess if the role can increase advancement, aiding career path planning. Furthermore, evaluate how the role contributes to broader leadership goals, ensuring each step is intentionally directed toward primary objectives.

Taking on a new position means embracing new possibilities. Connect current responsibilities with overarching goals, recognizing that every challenge and success as a physician leader contributes to future career ambitions. Maintaining awareness of this connection turns routine tasks into valuable experiences that propel forward. This mindset enhances leadership abilities and keeps the focus on ultimate goals, ensuring a fulfilling and impactful professional journey.

11. **Applying 1-Year Plan**: To be successful during the first year in academic medicine, it is wise to divide the year into three 4-month periods to monitor growth regularly. We recommend the following steps to achieve success during this crucial period:
    - **Start with the End in Mind**: It's always wise to measure the progress in terms of SMART goals. SMART goals are:
        - **Specific**: Clearly define what you want to achieve.
        - **Measurable**: Ensure that your progress can be tracked with quantifiable indicators.
        - **Achievable**: Set realistic goals that are within your capacity to accomplish.
        - **Relevant**: Align your goals with your broader objectives and values.
        - **Time-Bound**: Establish a clear timeline for achieving your goals.
        - **Write a Plan for the First Year as a Leader in a Medical Institution**: Creating a detailed plan outlining the year's objectives, strategies, and actions is advisable. This plan should include:
    - **Personal Transition Markers**: Regularly reflect on the adaptation to the new role and your personal growth.
        - **Content Learning Goals**: Identify the critical areas of knowledge and skills needed to acquire and outline how they should be achieved.
        - **Team Building Strategies**: Developing a plan for building strong, trustworthy teams and enhancing communication skills.
        - **Organizational Integration**: Understanding the organizational culture, building relationships at various levels, and finding ways to add value to the institution.

    By following these steps and regularly reviewing your progress, you can ensure a successful transition into your role in academic medicine.

Phase 2: Launching Phase (Months 0–4)

The launching phase is about making a strong, positive first impression and setting the tone of your leadership style. It is important to clearly articulate your vision and expectations to align with team and institution goals. It is also important to achieve early successes, the so-called quick wins or low-hanging fruit, to build momentum and confidence as a leader.

1. **Present as Leader**. Physician leaders must focus on being genuine leaders, not just managers. This journey should commence from day one, emphasizing setting clear goals, leading the team, and delivering results.

    - **Set a Clear Direction**: Physician leaders may not have all the answers, but they are courageous enough to search for them. As a renowned American business executive and author Jack Welch once said, "The best leaders don't have all the answers, but they do know how to ask the right questions" [10]. A leader must set a clear direction for themselves and their team, which involves defining a vision, planning the required actions to achieve it, and ensuring everyone is aware of their role in the process. In times of uncertainty, a leader's commitment to solving problems provides confidence and guidance.
    - **Bring People Together**: As physician leaders, it's crucial to remember that people are always observing and eager to understand. Effective leadership requires transparent communication. "Leadership is not about titles, positions, or flowcharts. It is about one life influencing another," as John C. Maxwell wisely stated [11]. Leaders share their goals, intentions, and expectations openly. By involving the team in decision-making and encouraging open discussions, the physician leaders build trust and ensure everyone strives toward the same objectives.
    - **Deliver Results**: It is crucial to deliver results promptly. Achieving quick wins helps to build momentum and prove the effectiveness of leadership skills. John C. Maxwell emphasized, "The secret of your success is determined by your daily agenda" [12]. Early accomplishments not only enhance morale but also establish credibility and set the stage for more substantial achievements down the road. Understanding the specific area of interest can lead to early success. Engaging in patient care within that particular area and generating research concepts can yield quick outcomes.

2. **Build Strong Team Relationships**: From the time of the start of the job, physician leaders should spend time building relationships with the people they work with, including nurses, trainees, clinic staff, peers, and seniors [13]. The purpose of these efforts is to break down barriers and build trust within the team. Leaders can create a more cohesive and collaborative working environment by fostering these relationships. This involves actively engaging with team members, understanding their perspectives, and showing genuine interest in their well-being and professional development.

    Leaders in this process should embody honesty, fairness, and enthusiasm. It is crucial to stay positive and provide value to team members to keep them motivated and inspired. Managing emotions, especially in stressful situations, is essential for setting a good example and making sound decisions. By following these guidelines, physician leaders can foster trust, respect, and teamwork, improving team performance and goal achievement [2].

3. **Manage Priorities**: Feeling overwhelmed in a new role, especially for physician leaders, is a common experience. The early stages of any position can present challenges that test one's resolve. However, a leader's passion helps them overcome these difficult times. By confronting challenges directly, leaders can grow and adapt. Acknowledging initial struggles and maintaining a positive outlook can significantly ease the transition and set the stage for future success. Spending time worrying about negative scenarios is counterproductive and can hinder progress. Leaders should embrace taking calculated risks and learning from their experiences. Leaders can overcome obstacles and propel their teams forward by focusing on potential opportunities and maintaining a proactive mindset. The ability to remain resilient and optimistic, especially in challenging times, is a crucial trait of effective leadership. This approach helps address current challenges and lays a foundation for sustained success and progress [8].
4. **Assess Success in the First 4 Months**: In the first 4 months of stepping into a new role as a physician leader, it's essential to prioritize rapid learning. This approach will help new leaders understand the new environment, meet role expectations, and prepare for unique challenges. Having a clear vision for the team is crucial for offering guidance and building trust in leadership. Confidence is vital as it empowers leaders to address challenges proactively and demonstrates readiness to lead. Patience is equally essential as leaders navigate the complexities of their role. It's important to remember that mistakes are part of the learning journey and provide valuable growth opportunities. Leaders view mistakes as steppingstones toward improvement. Building solid connections is critical to achieving success in the initial months. It's all about people and their interactions. Recognizing personal relationships within the team and fostering a collaborative environment will facilitate productive teamwork and communication. Establishing a support network with colleagues can offer essential advice and insights to enhance approaches and strategies. This support system can also provide emotional and professional backing, helping leaders stay resilient and committed to their goals. By focusing on these critical success factors, leaders can lay a solid foundation for their leadership journey and ensure a positive start in their new role.

   After 4 months, leaders must engage in self-reflection. This will start by assessing how they manage their time and energy, handle communication, and deal with challenges in their new role. Evaluate their team composition and performance and consider any necessary adjustments. Reflect on their alignment with their superiors and overall well-being to prevent burnout. By addressing these areas, leaders can gain valuable insights and make informed adjustments for continued success.

Phase 3: Momentum Phase (4–8 Months)

The momentum phase revolves around continuing to build on previous successes and maintaining enthusiasm, progress, and energy both for yourself and your team. It is also strategically a good time to consider introducing more significant changes and initiatives.

As leaders reach the 4–8-month mark of their first year, striving for excellence in leadership is crucial. This involves continuously working on personal growth and remaining committed to responsibilities. Leadership is a skill that evolves with time and requires continuous improvement. At this stage, leaders should seek feedback from colleagues, mentors, and team members to identify areas for growth and demonstrate a willingness to adapt and progress. By committing to becoming an exceptional leader, leaders will cultivate trust and loyalty within their team.

Understanding the importance of tackling challenges is crucial for achieving success. It is essential to face problems with a practical mindset, recognizing the situation rather than evading it. Leaders can create feasible solutions and make informed choices by addressing issues head-on. Leveraging the insights gained in recent months, leaders can implement required adjustments, such as refining strategies, reallocating resources, or reshaping team structures to better align with objectives. Showing flexibility and promptly addressing new challenges will improve leaders' effectiveness.

Investing in establishing connections is crucial at this moment. Cultivating and managing solid professional relationships can offer priceless assistance, resources, and opportunities. It's vital to allocate time for networking with individuals within and outside the company. These engagements may result in fresh partnerships, mentorship prospects, and increased recognition in your field. This stage is focused on creating momentum, aiding leaders in building the momentum necessary for long-term success.

By the end of the eighth month, reviewing and updating the plan for the first year is crucial. This process involves reflecting deeply on one's progress and the challenges encountered. Such reflection enables leaders to identify and implement any required adjustments to the plan. It is also an opportune moment to establish new objectives, refine strategies, and ensure these goals align with the division's objectives. Regularly reviewing and revising the plan will help leaders stay on track toward achieving long-term goals.

Phase 4: Consolidation Phase (8–12 Months)

The consolidation phase is crucial for physician leaders to prepare for a successful career long term. It allows for the stabilization of the department after any changes previously implemented in the last 8 months and allows new processes to be more fully implemented and integrated into the daily life of the team. You can take stock and make any adjustments needed to go forward and reinforce the desired culture and value within the team.

This final phase involves combining all the knowledge acquired over the past 8 months and aligning it with their long-term goals to achieve a successful career. During this phase, we recommend the following:

1. **Actively Ask for Feedback**: As a physician leader, seeking feedback rather than reassurance from the team and seniors is essential to develop and improve continuously. According to the well-known leadership educator and mentor Peter Drucker, "Effective feedback is not just about giving praise or criticism; it is about providing actionable insights that help people improve" [14]. Feedback provides valuable insights into one's performance, highlighting areas of strength and opportunities for growth. Engaging in open and constructive conversations with colleagues and mentors allows leaders to understand different perspectives and make informed adjustments to one's leadership approach. By actively seeking feedback, leaders demonstrate a commitment to personal and professional development, fostering a culture of continuous improvement within their team. Refer to the feedback chapter to grasp the basics of receiving feedback and the significance of breaking it down into actionable steps.
2. **Developing Resilience and Resourcefulness**: Physician leaders should prioritize developing resilience, which involves dedication, perseverance, a positive mindset, and the ability to recover from setbacks. Dedication keeps leaders focused on their goals despite obstacles, perseverance helps them conquer challenges, and a constructive outlook empowers them to address issues with hope. Resilience allows leaders to rebound from setbacks quickly, learn from failures, and keep moving forward, helping them navigate the demands of medical leadership. As Nelson Mandela said, "Do not judge me by my success; judge me by how many times I fell and got back up again" [15].

   Resourcefulness encompasses problem-solving, creativity, and adaptability as a leader encounters challenges that require innovative approaches. Being resourceful entails critical and creative thinking to surmount obstacles. Problem-solving abilities aid in pinpointing effective tactics, while creativity fosters thinking beyond conventional boundaries. Adaptability facilitates adjusting to changes and maintaining effectiveness across different scenarios. Developing resourcefulness prepares leaders to tackle various issues and guide their team adeptly through any circumstance.

   Leaders must focus on this phase to develop resilience and resourcefulness, ultimately determining their short- and long-term success.
3. **Building Connection with the Teams**: During this critical time, leaders need to stay connected with others. Building strong relationships is vital for successful teamwork and collaboration. Leaders should engage with their peers, value their viewpoints, and encourage development. By nurturing these connections, leaders establish a supportive community that aids in overcoming obstacles and reaching objectives. Furthermore, leaders ought to recognize their accomplishments. Self-motivation is crucial for sustaining confidence

and drive. They should commemorate achievements and advancements, reflecting on the beneficial influence being generated. Building a positive and strong emotional bond with the team is essential. This includes establishing trust, loyalty, and morale through empathy, celebrating achievements, and supporting during challenges.

As the first year wraps up, physician leaders must review their progress. They should reflect on their goals, assess their achievements, and pinpoint areas needing improvement. Evaluating the foundation set for the next 3–5 years and ensuring alignment with long-term success is essential. Considering stakeholder feedback is vital for meeting expectations.

Leaders must also consider how respected and trusted they are by their team, a key indicator of effective leadership. Evaluating performance against organizational goals is essential. Highlighting accomplishments and progress, both qualitatively and quantitatively, is critical to showcasing quick wins and identifying areas for improvement. Reflecting on past experiences can guide future approaches.

Record the Achievements and Lessons Learned

Leaders must reflect on their significant accomplishments with pride for what they have achieved. These successes are not just career milestones but also serve as guides for future endeavors. A leader must consider the changes they have made in the first year and how they have impacted their performance. Evaluating these adjustments, whether trying new tactics, enhancing communication, or refining team-building skills, can emphasize the significance of flexibility and continuous growth. By recording their triumphs and challenges, leaders create a comprehensive record of their progress that can influence their future decisions and plans.

Getting Ready for the Time Beyond the First Year

As physician leaders approach the end of their first year, preparing for steady-paced momentum is crucial. The initial period of rapid adjustment and intense learning has laid a solid foundation, and now it is time to build on that with a more consistent and sustainable approach. Setting a manageable pace allows for continued growth and development without the risk of burnout. Maintaining the established positive habits and routines and balancing the workload are essential to sustaining energy and enthusiasm over the long term.

Focusing on long-term success involves setting strategic goals that extend beyond immediate achievements. Start thinking about the next steps in the career and the broader impact to have within the organization. Develop a vision for where to be in the next 3–5 years and outline the steps needed. This could involve further professional development, taking on new challenges, or leading innovative projects. Long-term success is about building a legacy of positive change and continuous improvement. By keeping an eye on the bigger picture, efforts today can contribute to meaningful and lasting achievements in the future.

Conclusions

In the first year of transitioning to a leadership role in academic medicine, establishing a robust foundation is essential for immediate success and long-term career development. The first year is critical for setting the tone of the leader's tenure, establishing effective leadership styles, and aligning with the team and organizational mission. This period demands strategic planning and a proactive approach to integrate into the academic community, laying the groundwork for a reputable presence and influence within the organization.

The chapter offers a structured roadmap divided into four phases—preparation, launching, momentum, and consolidation. Each phase focuses on different aspects of transitioning, from letting go of past roles and building professional networks to managing personal and professional growth effectively. This structured approach helps minimize the overwhelming nature of the transition while maximizing the opportunities for leadership and personal development. Ultimately, the guidance aims to cultivate a legacy of innovation and leadership, ensuring that the efforts made in the first year pave the way for future achievements and career fulfillment.

Take-Home Points

- Maintain a balance between clinical duties and academic endeavors to build a solid foundation for future achievements.
- Establish strategic objectives and create a well-defined vision to steer the career path and coincide with organizational goals.
- Establish strong professional connections early on to help navigate the challenges of the role and boost career advancement.
- Implement a well-organized, step-by-step transition strategy to successfully navigate the obstacles of taking on new leadership positions.

References

1. Bennett RT. The light in the heart: inspirational thoughts for living your best life. Roy Bennett; 2021.
2. Watkins M. The first 90 days, updated and expanded: proven strategies for getting up to speed faster and smarter. Gen121; 2013.
3. BrainyQuotes. https://www.brainyquote.com/quotes/michael_j_fox_189302. Accessed 4 Jul 2024.
4. Covey SR. The 7 habits of highly effective people: powerful lessons in personal change. Free Press; 2004.
5. Sharma R. The greatness guide: 101 lessons for making what's good at work and in life even better. Harper Business; 2008.
6. Lencioni P. The five dysfunctions of a team: a leadership fable, 20th anniversary edition. Jossey-Bass; 2002.
7. Meyer J. Battlefield of the mind: winning the battle in your mind. Warner Faith; 2002.
8. O'Keeffe N. Your first 100 days: make maximum impact in your new role. FT Press; 2019.
9. QuoteFancy. https://quotefancy.com/quote/879654/Oprah-Winfrey-A-mentor-is-someone-who-allows-you-to-see-the-hope-inside-yourself-A-mentor.
10. Royse D. 10 Great Jack Welch quotes on leadership, developing talent and more. 2020. https://finance.yahoo.com/news/10-great-jack-welch-quotes-223010106.html?guccounter=1&guce_referrer=aHR0cHM6Ly93d3cuZ29vZ2xlLmNvbS8&guce_referrer_sig=AQAAAIVK2buIZZeHiuHkmfqju5TYDEudwTp5XsFvTXehxqiPRz8dpvBRntu18B-UlIUf-CD9uP2ZwNnGrbYIE02jM3J1Nwx27DYu-Kdh0POGE4vqzAJFZ8p9vTot4EZUCh7TQIuyTGDqZQpIIH1iQDzPZ6maXvO-Fa0EFv3n1ZEdrnMp#.
11. Maxwell JC. The 21 indispensable qualities of a leader: becoming the person others will want to follow. Thomas Nelson; 1999.
12. QuoteFancy. https://quotefancy.com/quote/841051/John-C-Maxwell-The-secret-of-your-success-is-determined-by-your-daily-agenda.
13. Theodore Roosevelt Center. https://theodorerooseveltcenter.org/Learn-About-TR/TR-Quotes?page=147#:~:text=The%20most%20important%20single%20ingredient,found%20to%20verify%20the%20attribution. Accessed 2024.
14. Ducker, P. The effective executive: The definitive guide to getting the right things done. Harper business. 2006.
15. Mandela: The Interview' Director: Ralph T. Niemeyer, 1994.

Chapter 3
Leadership Styles and Levels

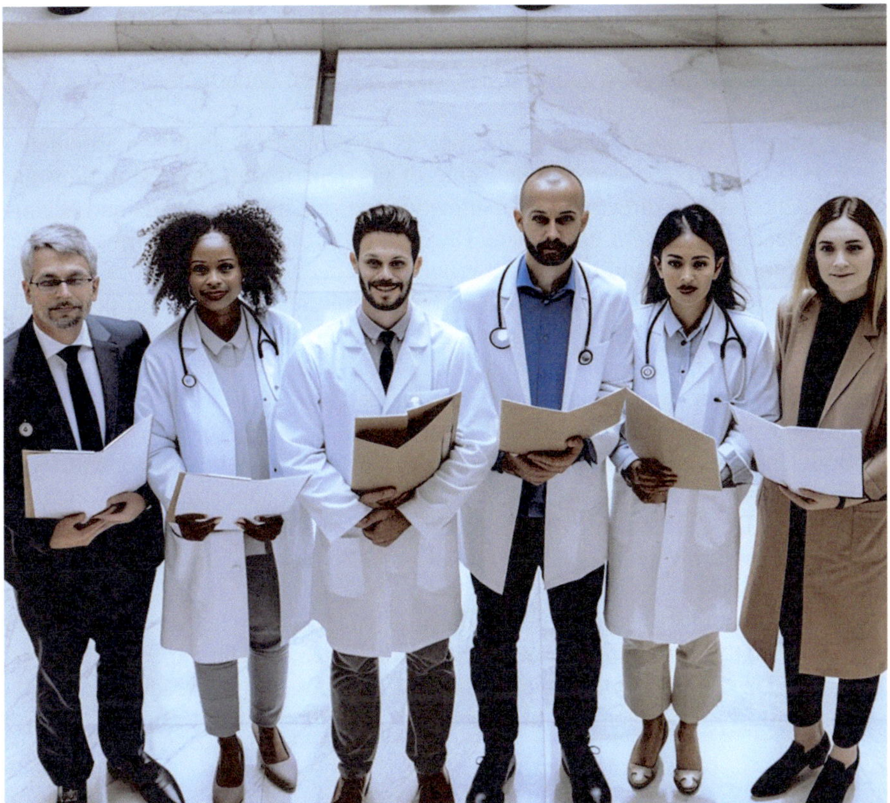

A. Djamali et al., *Emerging Leaders in Academic Medicine*,
https://doi.org/10.1007/978-3-031-80358-1_3

Case Presentation

Dr. Jones and Dr. Carter are emerging leaders in different departments at an academic medical center. Both are highly skilled and respected by their peers, but they exhibit distinctly different leadership styles, each reflecting their personalities and values.

Dr. Jones is known for his people-centered and collaborative approach to leadership. He believes in the power of teamwork and strives to create an inclusive environment where all voices are heard. His leadership style is participative; he actively seeks input from colleagues and staff when making decisions. Dr. Jones frequently organizes interdisciplinary meetings, encouraging open dialogue and fostering a sense of shared ownership over projects. This results in a high level of team cohesion, and his department experiences a lower rate of turnover and higher levels of engagement than national averages. This culture of collaboration fosters innovation and empowers the team to share ideas and take initiative. However, challenges can arise when quick, decisive action is needed or the issue under consideration is not one that allows for group input.

Dr. Carter is a task-oriented leader who is known for his ability to articulate a clear and compelling vision for the future of his department. He is ambitious and goal-oriented with a directive leadership style; he sets high standards and encourages his team to strive for excellence. Dr. Carter's strong sense of purpose is often enough to propel him and his team through challenges, although it does not allow for much input from the team along the way. This results in a high-performing department, and his ability to inspire and challenge his team yields significant achievements and recognitions. However, his result-oriented approach can lead to stress and burnout among team members who feel pressure to meet his high expectations and struggle with a lack of autonomy.

Both Dr. Jones and Dr. Carter demonstrate effective leadership, albeit in different ways. Dr. Jones excels in fostering a collaborative and supportive work environment, while Dr. Carter's singular vision drives his team to high achievement. Both leaders also must deal with potential fallout from their leadership styles, again albeit of different kinds.

This case study illustrates how differing leadership styles can impact team dynamics and outcomes in an academic medical center. The experiences of Dr. Jones and Dr. Carter highlight the importance of adaptability in leadership and the value of tailoring one's leadership approach to the situation and team.

Introduction

"Everything rises and falls on leadership." This powerful statement by the famous American writer and inspirational speaker, John C Maxwell, defines why understanding and practicing leadership is so essential for both the personal and professional growth of individuals and organizations [1]. Understanding leadership styles and levels is crucial for professional development in any industry, including health-care. It is essential to produce more effective physician leaders who better understand this complex health system.

Our default leadership style is the approach we feel most comfortable with when leading others toward our vision and goals and the style we usually revert to when under pressure. Knowing more about leadership styles helps us to avoid the common mistakes associated with each style. It is important to note that no leadership style is superior or inferior to another, and leaders must demonstrate essential mental, emotional, and cognitive abilities regardless of their default preferences. Moreover, a lack of personal integrity is the archenemy of leadership. Integrity in leaders implies being honest, dependable, and reliable. Leaders build their integrity from within and in the eyes of the people around them and act in accordance with their values.

Successful leaders understand their leadership style and the leadership styles of the people around them. Notably, they practice "dynamic leadership" and change their leadership style based on the situation. In John Maxwell's words, "The true measure of leadership is influence—nothing more, nothing less" [1].

Leadership Styles

Kurt Lewin, a German American psychologist, first defined leadership styles about seven decades ago [2]. There are several leadership styles, but the primary ones are autocratic, democratic, transformational, and laissez-faire leadership, based on whether one is people-oriented or task-oriented (Fig. 3.1):

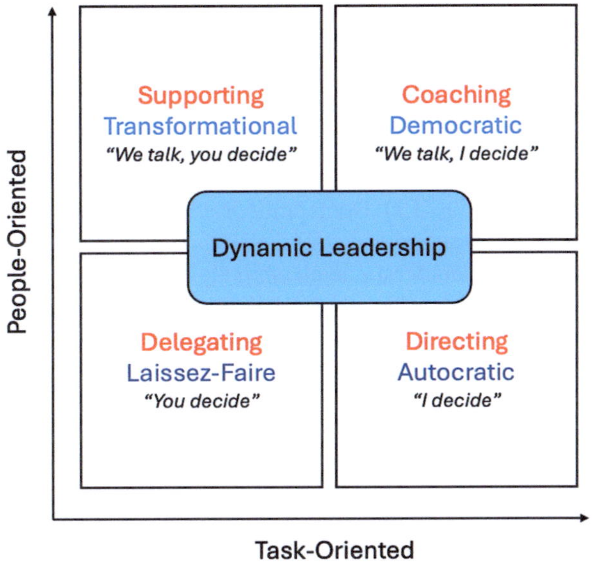

Fig. 3.1 Leadership styles based on whether one is people-oriented or task-oriented

Autocratic Leadership

Autocratic leadership focuses on the leader, who makes the decision without much input from the team (Fig. 3.1). Typically, autocratic leaders are task-oriented individuals who decide and then communicate with the team to execute the plan. It's a military style of leadership where the chain of command is maintained. In the healthcare system, it's when physician leaders make decisions without much consultation from the junior staff, nurses, or administrative staff.

Advantages of Autocratic Leadership

1. Decisions are often made at a fast pace, which can relieve the anxiety of the team members.
2. It improves performance in certain situations (for example, when a patient gets sick and quick decisions need to be made).
3. This leadership is sometimes needed in healthcare systems facing basic financial and administrative challenges.

Autocratic leadership should be used when quick decisions are needed to get things done. It can be highly beneficial in short-term choices and should be based on the context. For example, autocratic leadership may be needed if unprofessional behavior is noticed. It is unacceptable for physicians to access the medical file of patients they don't care for. Similarly, it is unacceptable to poorly manage clinical documentation and chart closures in patient care. However, this kind of leadership is not sustainable over the long term when you need to create buy-in and lead through change. For physician leaders, it's essential to promote a culture where every team member feels valued and has a role in making the final decision.

Democratic Leadership

Democratic leadership focuses on the team, with the decision-making shared across the group (Fig. 3.1). Democratic leaders focus on building relationships with an eye on job satisfaction and staff development. In the healthcare system, physician leaders with a democratic leadership style gather the opinions of all team members at the organizational level and daily work, even if they have the final word. This leadership style focuses on improving processes and systems rather than blaming individuals for failures.

Advantages of Democratic Leadership

1. There is a decreased risk of catastrophic failure as all the information is gathered before making the decisions. It's a shared decision, so every aspect of the decision is well thought out by the team members.
2. Shared decision-making creates buy-in and a feeling of ownership.
3. It increases collaboration between team members and generates a more reliable and comfortable work environment, ultimately improving team satisfaction.
4. Long-term democratic leadership encourages high performance.

Democratic leadership is beneficial at the organizational level and in daily work when the subordinates are experts, though achieving that can require extra effort. For example, a strategic planning retreat can help a new physician leader define the mission, vision, values, and strategic priorities for the team. During this exercise, expert members from the team gather and analyze the strengths, weaknesses, opportunities, and threats (SWOT analysis) for the group, and with the support of the leader, define the roadmap for the next 3–5 years. If led successfully, a democratic leader will influence the outcome and reap the benefits of the team's expertise while creating buy-in and commitment from the group.

Transformational Leadership

Transformational leaders are driven by change with a coaching style, as they perform their role so effectively that they gain the trust, respect, appreciation, and loyalty of the people who follow them. In its ideal form, transformational leadership creates valuable and positive change in the followers with the end goal of developing followers into leaders. Typically, the coach states "We talk, you decide" (Fig. 3.1). In healthcare, transformational leadership involves:

1. Setting clear and consistent goals.
2. Encouraging the team.
3. Leading through influence and charisma.
4. Modeling integrity.
5. Inspiring others to take on challenges.
6. Helping people to look beyond their interests.
7. Offering options to team members and helping them make informed decisions.

Advantages of Transformational Leadership

1. Through their passion and influence, transformational leaders communicate their vision well and get everyone on board.
2. Leaders can quickly analyze the situation and create a vision for the team for improvement and growth.

3. It helps followers build an environment to become future leaders.
4. It promotes a culture of integrity.
5. It helps teams look at the bigger picture and a road map to achieve the bigger goal.

Transformational leadership in healthcare is a powerful tool if used correctly. It helps physician leaders look beyond self-interest and provide inspiration and motivation to the members of the team. Integrity is the most critical component of transformational leadership. Here is an example of transformational leadership: consider you are working in a multidisciplinary team, caring for a patient with congestive heart failure. The first-year intern would like your advice as his senior resident regarding the management of diuretics prior to discharging the patient home. You can easily give the name of a drug and the dose, for example, furosemide 20 mg daily, taken orally, every morning. But you can also share your thoughts about options to use different diuretics, their relative side effects, the best ways to monitor for safety and efficacy, and let the intern make the decision after some thought. While the first approach is efficient and gets straight to the point, the second option has a long-lasting effect. It's the typical example of "Give a man a fish, and you feed him for a day; teach a man to fish and you feed him for a lifetime." This is ransformational/coaching style leadership.

Laissez-Faire Leadership

In a laissez-faire leadership style, the leader allows the team to self-direct (Fig. 3.1). In the healthcare system, laissez-faire leaders have an attitude of trust and reliance on their employees and the status quo. These leaders let their followers use their creativity, resources, and experience to help reach the bigger goal and vision of the physician leader. It's the opposite of autocratic leadership.

Advantages of Laissez-Faire Leadership

1. Personal growth and motivation: leaders trust their followers and allow them to grow and attain the skills they need.
2. Freedom of decision-making encourages innovation among the team members. Team members with more skills and experience need more freedom in how they work; this kind of leadership provides them with this opportunity.
3. With no micromanagement, team members can make faster decisions.

Laissez-faire leadership can only be successful if the team members are highly skilled and are motivated to achieve the shared goals. For example, your team members may be asking you whether they can work remotely for a period. Depending on their expertise, motivation, and kind of work, you may trust them to work remotely if the job gets done. You trust them and hold them accountable for the outcome, without micromanaging their day-to-day activity. This approach may work well for regulatory or administrative work, but it may not be feasible for clinicians that need to see patients in person.

Leadership Style of Successful Physician Leaders: The Concept of Dynamic Leadership

Physician leaders must be able to maintain integrity with their seniors, peers, and juniors and understand how to adapt their leadership style based on the situations and personalities involved to achieve their goals and vision. Autocratic and democratic leadership styles are more task-oriented, while transformational and laissez-faire leadership styles are more people-oriented. On a solid foundation of integrity, they develop a multidimensional or dynamic leadership style (Fig. 3.1). For example, they adopt an autocratic leadership style when urgent decisions are needed. For long-term success, they involve all the team members and adopt a democratic leadership style to assess every potential consequence of a decision and to give ownership of the long-term decisions to the team members. For the growth of the junior team members, the practice of transformational leadership is critical so that followers can grow into future leaders. When dealing with highly skilled followers, laissez-faire leadership is essential, giving the team members more confidence and practicing their skills.

Levels of Leadership

As mentioned earlier, it's essential for physician leaders in the academic healthcare system to understand the basics of leadership. A better understanding of the levels of leadership provides young leaders with information on where they stand and the roadmap to improve.

It is generally accepted that there are five levels of leadership, which provide an excellent road map for leaders to climb the leadership ladder gradually (Fig. 3.2). We will briefly describe those levels of leadership here and how applicable they are to physician leaders.

Level 1 Leadership: Position-Level Physician Leader

Level 1 leadership is the first rung of the leadership ladder: at this level, physician leaders are leaders due to their position. In the academic healthcare systems, we all start with a position. Even as a resident, fellow, or assistant professor, people around us and working for us follow us because of our position. There is nothing wrong with this level; however, stagnating on this level is a problem for someone with

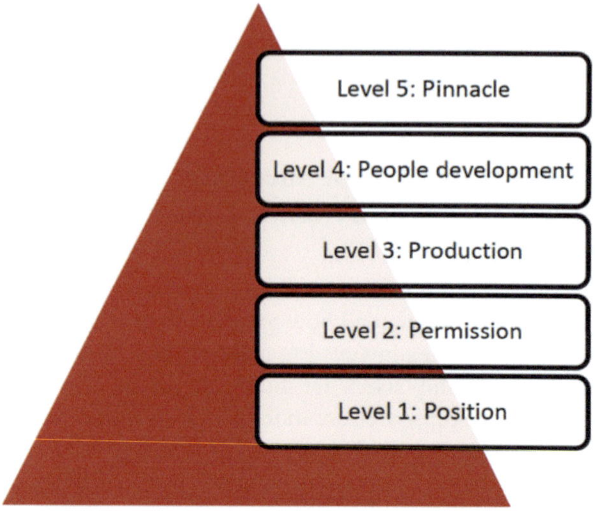

Fig. 3.2 Five levels of leadership. (Concept adopted from John Maxwell's five levels of leadership) [3]

higher leadership aspirations. Physician leaders should develop the skills to climb up from this level over time. It is critical to understand that this is the level to start from when starting a new job in any academic center. Authentic leadership is not about the position.

Tips to Reach the Next Level of Leadership

1. Display a high level of character and integrity. This builds trust and credibility, which are essential for effective leadership.
2. Define your values. Clear values guide decision-making and set a standard for the team.
3. Use your position to help people. Empowering others fosters a positive and productive work environment.
4. Develop an understanding of the people around you. Knowing your team's strengths and weaknesses, as well as needs enhances collaboration and performance.
5. Immerse yourself within the team. Active participation and engagement demonstrate commitment and inspire others.
6. Develop influence with the people. Influence enables leaders to motivate and guide their teams toward common goals.
7. Lead above, below, and across. Effective leadership requires managing relationships and responsibilities at all levels within the organization.

Level 2 Leadership: Permission-Level Physician Leader

The second level of leadership is the permission level of leadership. After building meaningful relationships with team members, the people around them follow the physician leaders not because of their position but because of their charisma and vision.

Physician leaders at this level are great with communication and always offer help when able. With their proven integrity and high values, people trust them. John Maxwell said, "We have to touch people's hearts before we ask for their hand."

Tips to Reach the Next Level of Leadership

1. Develop a connection with people that goes beyond just communication; this fosters trust and loyalty, which are essential for effective leadership.
2. Invest in people to grow them; supporting others' development builds a stronger, more capable team.
3. Always put people's growing interests first; prioritizing team members' growth enhances their engagement and helps performance.
4. Develop a clear goal and vision that followers can see. A clear vision inspires and aligns the team toward common objectives.
5. Develop a culture of respect. Respectful environments promote collaboration and reduce conflicts.
6. Develop a culture of trust. Trust encourages open communication and risk-taking, leading to innovation and growth.
7. Be a source of encouragement for the team. Encouragement boosts morale and motivates the team to achieve their best.
8. Deploy the team to areas of their interests and strengths. Aligning the roles with strengths maximizes productivity and job satisfaction.

Level 3 Leadership: Production-Level Physician Leader

This is the level of leadership where physician leaders display their true abilities and potential, demonstrating their ability to make things happen despite difficulties. They not only produce results individually but also help team members produce results. This level of leadership attracts others and models how to be more productive and influential members of the team. Reaching this leadership level adds credibility to the leaders, who become role models for others struggling with level 1 leadership.

Physician leaders at this level develop a certain degree of momentum, which helps them to solve several problems. In John Maxwell's words, "Momentum is a leader's best friend." This degree of momentum is needed to solve several complicated issues.

Tips to Reach the Next Level of Leadership

1. Develop a better understanding of your abilities. Self-awareness allows leaders to leverage strengths and address and improve weaknesses.
2. Stay clear in your vision and mission. Clarity in vision and mission ensures consistent and focused leadership.
3. Continue to inspire people at levels 1 and 2. Inspiring other junior leaders fosters a culture of leadership and growth across the organization.
4. Continue to help people be more productive and achieve personal growth. Supporting others' productivity and growth enhances overall team performance and morale.
5. Celebrate the small successes with the team. Recognizing achievements boosts morale and can motivate continued work.
6. Know how to prioritize to get a high-yield return. Effective prioritization maximizes resource utilization and impact.
7. Maintain the momentum of achievements. Sustaining momentum keeps the team motivated and focused on continued success and improvements.

Level 4 Leadership: People Development-Level Physician Leader

At this leadership level, physician leaders change themselves from producers to developers. After reaching this level, they better understand team members' potential, strengths, and weaknesses and have a much more powerful and significant impact on the people around them. Physician leaders at this level spend their energy thinking about how to grow the other team members. By working on the growth of all the team members, the leaders ensure the sustained growth of the team. Leaders recruit the best people and know where to place them for their personal growth and the growth of the whole team. They empower other people so they can also lead and succeed. They work as a role model for their entire team. In Ralph Nadar's words, "The function of leadership is to produce more leaders, not more followers." Metaphorically, these leaders are a rising tide; they lift all the ships.

Tips to Reach the Next Level of Leadership

1. Keep working on personal development. Continuous self-improvement enhances your skills and adaptability as a leader.
2. Don't let inner insecurities take over. Overcoming insecurities builds confidence and resilience, both of which are essential for effective leadership.
3. Keep working on maximizing team members' strengths and success. Focusing on team members' strengths drives team achievement and growth.

4. Keep yourself approachable to people. Approachability fosters open communication and trust within the team.
5. Continue to be a role model for the team. Leading by example inspires and motivates others to emulate positive behavior and attitude.

Level 5 Leadership: Pinnacle-Level Physician Leader

Level 5 is the highest level of leadership. Physician leaders at this level help others to reach level 4 leadership. Leaders at this level make room for others to reach the top. They work on people's strengths and provide them with a platform where they can perform their best. They have an attitude of giving away the power instead of holding onto it. They mentor people on other levels of leadership to become level 5 leaders. They always have a plan for their succession and leave a positive legacy behind them. In John Adam's words, "If your actions inspire others to dream more, learn more, do more, and become more, you are a leader."

The Following Traits Define a Level 5 Leader

1. Strong personal humility. Humility allows leaders to acknowledge their limitations and value others' contributions. Humility is not thinking less of yourself but rather thinking of yourself less often.
2. Incredibly driven and ambitious. Ambition fuels a leader's pursuit of goals and inspires others to strive to do their best.
3. High level of self-awareness. Self-awareness enables leaders to understand their impact on others and make informed decisions.
4. Incredibly emotionally intelligent. Emotional intelligence helps leaders manage relationships and navigate social complexities effectively and successfully.
5. Always putting the needs of others above their own. Leaders who do this foster a supportive and collaborative environment.
6. Displaying a high level of integrity. Integrity builds trust and sets an ethical standard for the team.
7. Proven ability to develop teams. Developing teams enhances collective skills and drives organizational success.
8. Excellent at maintaining a connection with the team, which is superior to just communication. Leaders who cultivate deeper connections with their team members foster loyalty and a strong team dynamic.

Tips to Maintain a Level 5 Leadership

1. Maintain focus. Staying focused ensures that leaders can effectively prioritize tasks and continue to achieve their goals. Focus also helps fuel the motivation to continue the hard work of leadership.
2. Remain humble. Humility allows leaders to stay grounded and open to feedback, fostering continuous improvement.
3. Remain teachable. A growth mindset ensures that leaders continue their personal growth and allows them to learn new information in a highly competitive and fast-paced environment and adapt accordingly to continue to achieve success.
4. Stay with people and don't let their stature push others away. Being approachable and inclusive strengthens cohesion and trust in already existing teams and helps invite others to contribute ideas and solutions to achieve goals.
5. Create room for other people to come to the top levels of leadership. Empowering others to rise fosters a culture of growth for all and also helps in succession planning for leaders when it is time to leave an organization.
6. Develop and invest in making other level 5 leaders. Investing in others leadership development at the highest levels ensures the sustainability and success of the organization.

The following points are essential to understanding the leadership levels (Fig. 3.3):

1. As junior faculty or trainee, we are at a different leadership level than the people we interact with. We need seniors to be our mentors. We need to help juniors advance in their leadership levels and peers to help them through the process.
2. Emerging physician leaders may start from level 1 when they start a new job.

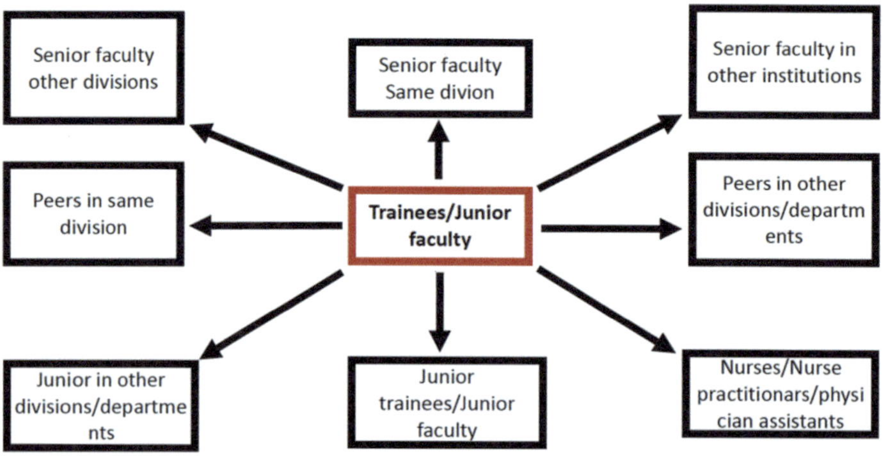

Fig. 3.3 An example of managing up, down, and across in academic leadership

3. As we advance on the leadership ladder, we must keep holding the previous leadership levels. For example, a level 5 leader would be retaining all other levels of leadership as well.
4. It is essential to recognize our leadership level and the leadership level of the people around us, as it provides us with a roadmap to climb the leadership ladder.

Leadership Vs. Management

Both leaders and managers are essential for the success of any organization. However, it is necessary to understand the difference between the two. In Peter Drucker's words, "Management is doing things right; leadership is doing the right things."

The distinction between managers and leaders lies not in job titles but in the execution of leadership responsibilities (Table 3.1). Irrespective of their hierarchical level, managers who effectively shoulder the responsibilities of leadership, such as offering inspiration, guidance, and crafting a vision for their subordinates, seamlessly transition into the realm of true leaders. It is a paradigm shift from merely overseeing tasks to actively inspiring and fostering growth among team members. Crucially, leadership transcends the confines of positional authority. It is a dynamic process deeply rooted in relationship building. Exceptional leaders understand that their influence is not derived solely from their title but from the quality of connections they forge with the people around them. This relational foundation becomes the bedrock upon which transformative leadership is built.

The essence of great leadership lies in the nuanced ability to comprehend the unique needs of individuals within the team. It involves delving into what they value, understanding their perspectives, and appreciating the diverse ways in which they perceive the world. Armed with this empathetic understanding, leaders guide their team members toward a shared vision that aligns with both organizational goals and individual aspirations.

Table 3.1 Basic differences between leaders and managers

Leaders	Managers
Leaders create positive change through their vision	Managers perform preplanned tasks
Leaders are people-oriented	Managers are task-oriented
Leaders have nothing to do with titles	Managers hold titles and subordinates who work for them
Leaders build influence	Managers have positional authority over the people
Leaders take initiatives	Managers follow orders
Leaders connect with people	Managers communicate with people
Leaders provide guidance	Managers micromanage

In the intricate dance of leadership, the ability to build relationships becomes a potent force for cohesion and collaboration. Great leaders are adept at creating an environment where individuals feel heard, valued, and understood. This fosters a sense of belonging and commitment, transcending the transactional aspects of management. Consistency is the hallmark of great leadership. Demonstrating an unwavering commitment to understanding the needs of the team and actively working toward a shared vision cements the leader's influence. It is this consistency that breeds trust, a cornerstone of effective leadership.

Leadership Competencies

While there are many institution- or health system-specific metrics, many are more universal and focus on leveraging individual strengths, fostering engagement, and driving performance. Per Gallup [4], the workplace consulting and global research experts, there are seven benchmark leadership competencies that you are most likely to be evaluated on as a leader.

1. **Build Relationships**: Strong interpersonal skills are crucial for leaders to build trust, collaborate effectively, and manage conflicts within their teams. When leaders build strong relationships, they create trust among team members, enhancing collaboration and productivity. Good relationships facilitate open communication, allowing leaders to better understand their team's abilities, perspectives, and challenges. Strong relationships encourage collaboration, as trust and respect lead to more effective teamwork and better outcomes. Leaders who invest in relationships inspire loyalty, with team members more likely to stay committed and engaged when they feel valued. Understanding team dynamics and individual strengths enables leaders to make informed decisions that benefit everyone. Collaborative relationships foster creativity and innovation, as people feel comfortable sharing ideas, leading to organizational success. Engaged employees are more productive, and building relationships shows that their well-being matters, increasing engagement levels. Teams with strong relationships can tackle challenges more effectively, benefiting from diverse perspectives and mutual trust. In summary, relationship building is essential for successful leadership, especially in today's digital economy where collaboration and adaptability are critical.
2. **Develop People**: Developing people is a key aspect of great leadership. Great leaders invest in the growth and development of their team members by providing coaching, feedback, and opportunities for advancement. Leadership development programs refine existing skills and introduce new strategies, enabling leaders to motivate, inspire, and guide their teams more effectively. These programs also hone a leader's ability to make informed decisions by teaching them to analyze situations, weigh options, and align choices with their vision. Understanding one's strengths, weaknesses, and growth opportunities allows

leaders to lead authentically and connect with their teams on a deeper level. Investing in leadership development fosters an environment where collaboration flourishes, boosting team morale and driving success. As a leader, it is your responsibility to develop others, empowering them to reach their full potential and contribute to the organization's mission. Good leaders respect individual uniqueness, draw out the best in people, and inspire purposeful teamwork.

3. **Lead Change**: Leading change is a crucial skill for effective leaders. They can create and communicate a compelling vision and purpose that inspires and aligns their team or organization. Change is inevitable in business, and leaders who embrace adaptability and resilience help their teams weather unexpected crises, market shifts, and organizational changes. Effective change management prevents low morale among employees, whether it's during mergers, acquisitions, or routine events, ensuring a positive experience for both staff and customers. Strong leadership during change eases worries, encourages communication, and addresses uncertainty, fostering a supportive environment where teams can adapt and thrive. Remember, change isn't just about reacting—it's about leading proactively to shape a better future for your team and organization.
4. **Inspire Others**: Inspiring others is a key trait of effective leaders. They are willing to take risks and make bold decisions when necessary, adapting to changing circumstances, handling stress, and bouncing back from setbacks. An inspiring leader has a clear vision and motivates others to work toward the same goal. By being on the front lines, they maximize people's potential, helping them get the most out of themselves. Inspiration builds trust and motivation, leading to better collaboration, stronger teamwork, and personal development. Inspiring leaders uplift morale, even during challenging times, providing structure and stimulus to steer the organizational ship toward success. As a leader, your ability to inspire creates a positive ripple effect throughout your team and organization.
5. **Think Critically**: Leaders should be able to think long term, understand market dynamics, and make informed decisions that position their team or organization for future success. Critical thinking allows leaders to anticipate potential challenges and devise strategies to overcome them, fostering a culture of continuous learning and improvement. A leader with critical thinking skills can understand the logical connections between ideas, identify the relevance and importance of arguments, detect inconsistencies or mistakes in reasoning, and make proper decisions. Leaders who develop critical thinking can rise above biases and assumptions that often hinder decision-making. By recognizing assumptions, evaluating arguments, and drawing informed conclusions, they enhance their decision-making ability. In today's complex and fast-paced world, critical thinking empowers leaders to navigate uncertainty and lead effectively.
6. **Communicate Clearly**: The ability to influence others and communicate clearly and persuasively is essential for leaders to gain buy-in and drive initiatives forward. Good communication is a key characteristic of successful leaders, essential for expressing ideas, sharing information, and achieving results through others. Being honest and sincere builds trust, as authenticity resonates with people. Avoiding corporate jargon and letting your true self shine through makes you

more relatable. Being present and visible, rather than hiding behind emails, helps you connect consistently with your team and stakeholders, reinforcing your leadership style. Great communicators are also active listeners, understanding others' perspectives, fostering trust, and aligning goals. Clear communication fosters collaboration, trust, and a shared vision, which are crucial for effective leadership.

7. **Create Accountability**: Leaders must demonstrate their accountability to their team and those above and below them in the organizational system. When leaders foster accountability, they build a culture of trust and responsibility. Clear expectations and constructive feedback enhance team performance, as accountable employees take initiative, demonstrate commitment, and work toward common objectives. This leads to increased productivity and improved performance. Accountability ensures that tasks are completed efficiently, contributing to successful project execution. A workplace that values accountability fosters greater commitment and employee happiness, resulting in lower turnover rates. In summary, accountable leaders empower their teams, drive results, and create a positive work environment.

Conclusion

The true essence of leadership lies not in titles or positions but in the art of relationship building and the ability to understand and guide individuals toward a collective vision. When managers embrace these principles of dynamic leadership styles and leadership levels, they evolve into leaders who inspire, empower, and foster a collaborative spirit within their teams.

Take-Home Points

- Understanding leadership styles and levels is essential for the professional growth of physician leaders.
- Successful physician leaders adopt a multidimensional dynamic leadership style where they can take on a leadership style as needed for the situation and the personalities.
- Successful physician leaders understand the leadership ladder and gradually climb to attain level 5 leadership.
- Successful physician leaders clearly understand the differences between leaders and managers and adapt to be a leader.

References

1. Maxwell JC. The 21 irrefutable laws of leadership. 2nd ed. HarperCollins Leadership; 2022.
2. Partners LP. Lewin's leadership theory explained. 2022. https://leadershipandperformance.com.au/leadership-development/lewins-leadership-theory-explained/. Accessed 6 Dec 2023.
3. Maxwell JC. The 5 levels of leadership: proven steps to maximize your potential. Hachette Book Group; 2011.
4. Gallup Corporation. 7 Expectations for transformational leaders. Gallup; 2021.

Chapter 4
Diversity, Equity, Inclusion, and Justice (DEIJ) in Academic Medicine

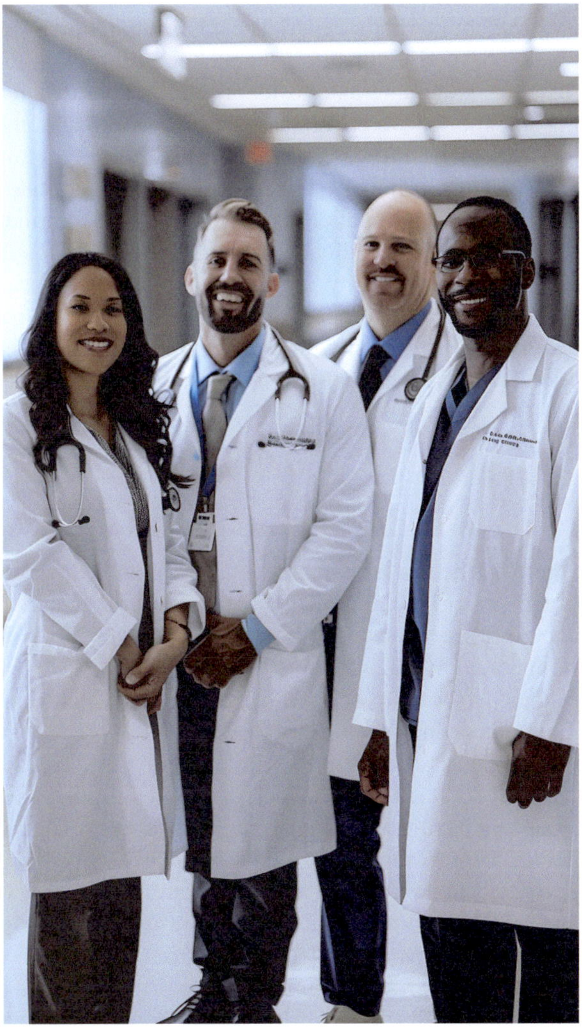

A. Djamali et al., *Emerging Leaders in Academic Medicine*,
https://doi.org/10.1007/978-3-031-80358-1_4

Case Presentation

Dr. Smith is a senior physician who leads a diverse team of medical residents. Despite being well meaning and committed to diversity, Dr. Smith's unconscious biases affect his interactions with his team and can impact his trainees in pernicious ways. During morning rounds, he often directs complex clinical questions to male residents as he assumes they have a stronger grasp of the materials. He directs fewer challenging questions to female residents and often assigns them basic tasks as he assumes they will be better at them. Dr. Smith's bias, however unconscious, can lead to lasting long-term career effects as they may miss out on critical learning experiences their male counterparts experience. Over time the residents themselves internalize this behavior, and the male residents begin to look at their female colleagues as less capable, and the female residents doubt their own abilities as well.

Dr. Johnson is an experienced physician who also works with this team of residents; they review a case where a Black patient presents with symptoms that suggest a complex condition. Unconsciously, Dr. Johnson downplays the severity of the symptoms and attributes them to patient behavior like non-compliance or lifestyle choices without considering the medical diagnoses that could account for all symptoms. This conclusion, influenced by unconscious racial bias, leads to a delayed diagnosis and a sub-optimum patient outcome. Moreover, it reinforces unconscious bias in the residents she is working with and sets the tone that it is okay to make general assumptions about patients based on factors like race, gender, or class.

Introduction

In recent years, there has been a growing recognition of and conversation around the pervasiveness of racism and social injustice within medical centers. With increased awareness of racial injustice in society, there is now a focus on the impact of racial bias in academic medicine. Organizations like the American Medical Association have increased their efforts to support diversity and inclusion in medicine. Nonetheless, despite these initiatives, the presence of Latino and Native American faculty in academic medical centers in the United States has seen a slight rise from 7% to 8% over the last 20 years [1]. The lack of progress in this area highlights the ongoing difficulties that healthcare must overcome to address social inequalities.

Academic medical centers must have a diverse faculty to meet their educational, clinical, and research objectives as well as provide culturally sensitive and inclusive healthcare. By including individuals from underrepresented groups, medical institutions can better cater to a diverse patient population and enhance the quality of medical education and research. Additionally, promoting equity and inclusiveness is vital for any healthcare organization. Unfortunately, there is a noticeable shortage of underrepresented minorities in leadership positions within academic medical centers despite the evident benefits of diversity [2]. Furthermore, even in cases where organizations have made strides in promoting diversity, there is still a lack of an inclusive and equitable culture.

When young doctors step into a fresh role in the healthcare sector, they must possess clinical skills and grasp organizational dynamics, patient care, and societal impacts. Physician leaders should understand the importance of and promote diversity, equity, and inclusion within their teams. They should also strive to address unconscious biases within themselves and their team. It is vital to raise awareness about these matters in all organizations, including medical schools. In this chapter, we will explore the importance of recognizing and addressing unconscious bias, how racism affects academic medicine, and the role of physician leaders in proactively addressing these issues. Medical institutions can move toward establishing a fairer and more inclusive healthcare system by comprehending and actively addressing these challenges.

Recognizing Pervasive Types of Bias

Understanding the different types of bias that commonly occur in academic medical settings is important for many reasons. Biases can lead to unfair treatment, discrimination, or favoritism. Recognizing biases helps ensure that all team members are treated equitably, regardless of their background, gender, race, or other characteristics. Biases can hinder diversity and inclusion efforts by creating barriers for underrepresented groups. Understanding biases helps in creating more inclusive hiring practices, promotions, workplaces, and patient policies. Biases can also cause misunderstandings, miscommunications, and conflicts. Recognizing these biases can help prevent and resolve conflicts by promoting empathy and understanding. Reduced workplace conflict leads to a more harmonious and collaborative work environment. Many forms of bias, such as those related to race, gender, and age, lead to discrimination, which is illegal and unethical. Being aware of biases helps leaders and organizations avoid legal issues and maintain ethical standards, protecting the company's reputation and reducing the risk of lawsuits.

A fair workplace fosters trust, respect, and a positive organizational culture. Biases can also cloud judgment and lead to poor decision-making. By being aware of biases, individuals and teams can make more rational, objective, and informed decisions. Better decision-making can in turn improve patient outcomes, improve business outcomes, productivity, and employee satisfaction. Biases can also lead to groupthink, where alternative ideas are not considered. By recognizing and addressing biases, organizations can create an environment where diverse ideas are welcomed and valued. This, then, can drive more innovative solutions and creativity in problem-solving.

Understanding biases allows individuals to reflect on their own behavior and attitudes, promoting personal growth and development. This self-awareness can lead to better interpersonal skills, leadership qualities, and a more supportive work environment. A workplace that actively works to minimize biases promotes a culture of inclusion, respect, and open-mindedness. A positive organizational culture attracts top talent, enhances employee satisfaction, and supports overall success.

Leaders who are aware of their own biases are better equipped to lead ethically and set an example for others. Ethical leadership promotes a healthy workplace, fosters trust, and guides the team in making principled decisions.

- **Confirmation Bias**: Clinicians may give more weight to information that confirms their preconceptions about a patient while disregarding or downplaying any evidence that contradicts these assumptions. This can lead to misdiagnosis or inappropriate treatment plans. Alternatively, emerging leaders may have a confirmation bias to recruit another physician of the same color, culture, or background as themselves, instead of someone from another organization, even if the latter is more competent.
- **Anchoring Bias**: This occurs when a clinician relies too heavily on the first piece of information they receive about a patient (the "anchor"), which can skew subsequent decision-making. Even as new information is made available, an anchoring bias can make it difficult for a clinician to move on from this anchor.
- **Recency or Dramatic Bias**: The tendency to overestimate the likelihood of events based on their availability in memory, often because they are recent or dramatic. This can lead providers to over-diagnose a condition they recently encountered or one that had a dramatic outcome, regardless of its actual prevalence.
- **Overconfidence Bias**: The tendency to overestimate one's own clinical judgment or abilities. This can lead to errors in diagnosis, treatment, or patient management when it leads physicians to dismiss alternate opinions or new information.
- **Attribution Bias**: The tendency to attribute patients' behavior to their character or personal choices rather than considering external factors. A doctor might assume a patient's symptoms are due to lifestyle choices rather than exploring other potential causes.

These biases are often unconscious and can occur despite the best intentions of healthcare providers. Recognizing and addressing these biases is crucial for improving patient care and reducing disparities in health outcomes.

Unraveling the Complexities of Unconscious Bias

Unconscious bias is a subtle yet pervasive force that shapes our perceptions, interactions, and decisions without our explicit awareness. Author of Everyday Bias: Identifying and Navigating Unconscious Judgements, Howard Ross, said, "Most unconscious bias is caused by well-intended people with blind spots" [3]. "Unconscious bias includes any assumption that is inaccurate," said Laura Castillo-Page, AAMC senior director [3]. These biases are difficult to recognize because they operate silently, deeply embedded within the subconscious layers of our minds, affecting our judgments and actions in ways we may not readily detect.

The human brain is structured to facilitate and resist the management of unconscious bias. It consists of ancient and modern components that handle different functions. The older part, located within the limbic system, is responsible for automatic processing and tends to rely on entrenched patterns of thinking and reacting. This part of the brain helps make quick decisions based on past experiences and deep-seated patterns, which can, unfortunately, include biased and prejudiced views. On the other hand, the modern brain, particularly the cortex, is equipped with the capacity for critical thinking and rational analysis. This part of the brain enables us to evaluate situations, consider various outcomes, and make well-thought-out decisions. However, leveraging the full capabilities of the cortex requires conscious effort and intentionality—it does not automatically take precedence over the more instinctive reactions of the limbic system [4].

For physician leaders, the implications of unconscious bias are significant in all aspects of their position, and therefore awareness and proactive management of these biases are crucial. Leaders must actively recognize their own biases and challenge them rigorously to ensure that they do not negatively impact their professional responsibilities. According to the renowned leadership coach Brene Brown, influential leaders acknowledge their biases and continuously try to confront and conquer them, thus establishing a benchmark for others to emulate [5]. This involves constantly seeking education on bias, engaging in self-reflection, and fostering an environment where diversity and inclusion are practiced and valued.

Moreover, replacing outdated and biased thinking patterns with fair and inclusive frameworks is essential. By critically examining their thoughts and adopting open-minded perspectives, physician leaders can lead by example, promoting a healthcare culture that advances fairness, equality, and respect for all patients and staff. Doing so improves the quality of care and contributes to a more equitable healthcare system.

Biases in the Clinical Setting

All the examples provided below speak about the impact these biases have on patients in clinical practice.

- **Racial/Ethnic Bias**: Clinicians may unconsciously assume certain characteristics or behaviors based on a patient's race or ethnicity, leading to disparities in diagnosis, treatment, and pain management. For example, Black and Hispanic patients often receive less pain medication compared to white patients. This can also be seen as language bias with patients who do not speak the dominant language or have limited health literacy. They may be perceived as less compliant or intelligent, leading to less engagement by healthcare providers.
- **Gender Bias**: Women may have their symptoms dismissed or downplayed, particularly in conditions like heart disease where symptoms can differ from those seen in men, or in gynecological conditions where there is no point of comparison with men. Gender bias can also lead to assumptions about a patient's mental health or emotional state, affecting the quality and amount of care provided.

- **Age Bias**: Older adults may be treated less aggressively for certain conditions, with assumptions made about their quality of life or potential for recovery. Conversely, younger patients might be perceived as more resilient, leading to under-treatment of serious conditions.
- **Weight Bias**: Patients with obesity often face stigma and may have their health concerns attributed solely to their weight, leading to missed diagnoses or less comprehensive and compassionate care. This bias can and frequently does discourage obese patients from seeking medical care altogether.
- **Socioeconomic Bias**: Assumptions about patient's socioeconomic status can influence how clinicians perceive their ability to adhere to treatment plans, afford medications, or understand medical instructions. This potentially results in clinicians putting forth less effort to explain or offer comprehensive care.
- **LGBTQIA+ Bias**: LBGTQIA+ individuals may experience assumptions about their sexual practices, health risks, or gender identity, which can lead to inadequate or inappropriate care. This bias can also create a lack of trust between a patient and provider, impacting overall health outcomes.
- **Disability Bias**: Patients with disabilities might be perceived as having a lower quality of life, leading to less aggressive treatment or different assumptions about their health needs. This bias can be seen with patients who have physical, intellectual, or psychiatric disabilities.

How Bias Impacts Healthcare Teams

Healthcare professionals who face these bias challenges find that it limits their career growth, with assumptions about their capabilities leading to fewer opportunities for promotion, training, or leadership roles. Bias may lead to the underestimation of a disabled team member's abilities, resulting in them being assigned less challenging or lower-responsibility tasks, which can stifle professional development. They may be excluded from certain activities, discussions, or social events—due to either physical or social barriers—which can lead to feelings of isolation. Conversely, sometimes team members might be included in teams only to meet diversity requirements (tokenism) without being genuinely included or valued. Bias can create a hostile work environment where marginalized team members might face microaggressions, derogatory remarks, or a lack of support from colleagues and leadership. Bias may lead to a lack of reasonable accommodation being provided, making it difficult for a team member to perform their duties effectively. Constantly facing bias or needing to advocate for themselves can lead to increased stress and burnout among marginalized healthcare workers. Feeling undervalued or discriminated against can reduce job satisfaction, potentially leading to high turnover rates. When team members are undervalued or excluded, teams miss out on diverse perspectives that can drive innovation, problem solving, and empathy in patient care. If bias prevents diverse trainees from accessing further education and training, the entire team may miss out on knowledge and skills they could have contributed.

Impact of Unconscious Bias in Academic Medicine

Several studies have shown that racism, discrimination, and inequity are significant problems in academic medicine [1, 6, 7].

- **Job Dissatisfaction**: The absence of diversity, equity, and inclusion is a significant contributor to job dissatisfaction. In a survey conducted by Price et al. at Johns Hopkins University, non-tenured physicians shared their belief that race, foreign-born status, and gender can lead to bias and unequal opportunities in the workplace. Minority and foreign-born faculty reported experiencing disparities in recruitment and promotion while facing inadequate retention efforts and a lack of mentorship that hindered their success and overall job satisfaction [8]. According to another study, underrepresented faculty members in academic medical centers often must continuously demonstrate their value, worth, and abilities [9], thus diverting their energies from more productive activities.
  It is also well documented that in academic medical centers, underrepresented minorities also face disparity in promotions [9–11]. As a result, under-represented minorities are frequently found in junior faculty compared to higher leadership positions [1].
- **Dysfunctional Teams**: A high-performance team is essential in the healthcare system, leading to better patient care and promoting staff well-being. A high-performance team comprises individuals who work together toward a common goal and are highly collaborative and innovative. These teams thrive in environments where appreciation and encouragement are valued, creating a culture of mutual respect and cooperation [12]. By recognizing and appreciating each team member's contributions, organizations can create an atmosphere leading to exceptional patient care outcomes.
  Unconscious biases among team members can harm team dynamics and hinder their ability to work effectively. These biases can lead to microaggressions that damage trust and communication among colleagues. This can result in disengagement and lack of cooperation, ultimately impacting the quality of care for patients. Physician leaders must address and reduce these biases to create a supportive and inclusive environment where all team members can contribute to their fullest potential.
- **Poor Patient Care**: Unconscious bias can harm patient care. It can manifest as a communication breakdown between physicians, patients, and other team members involved in the patient's care, or as assumption-making about a patient's pain capacity based on their race or gender. This can result in diagnostic uncertainty, negative clinical interactions, and less patient-centeredness [13].
- **Effect on Recruitment and Retention**: Unconscious bias presents significant challenges within the healthcare sector, particularly affecting current physicians and potential new hires. Physicians who detect bias in their workplace often feel undervalued and misunderstood, which can lead them to seek employment elsewhere rather than stay long term at an institution. Similarly, potential employees who sense bias during recruitment are less likely to accept job offers, deterred by

their perceived lack of inclusivity. These dynamics can severely impact crucial hiring decisions, harming the health organization's ability to maintain a stable, engaged, diverse workforce. Such turnover disrupts continuity of care and affects the institution's overall performance and financial health.

According to research by Talent Innovation, employees in large organizations who perceive bias are three times more likely to disengage from their work. This disengagement can manifest as a lack of motivation and a decrease in job performance, with employees over two times more likely to withhold innovative ideas, further stifling organizational growth and improvement. The desire for a diverse and inclusive workplace is a critical factor in job satisfaction for employees and potential hires [14]. Regrettably, many health organizations miss opportunities to enhance their teams with various perspectives by failing to recruit and hire new physicians from diverse backgrounds. This not only limits the cultural competency of the healthcare team but also restricts the organization's ability to connect with and effectively treat a diverse patient population.

Strategies to Fight Unconscious Bias in Academic Medical Centers

Healthcare organizations and physician leaders have a shared responsibility to combat unconscious bias. As physician leaders, we suggest strategies to reduce unconscious bias and create an inclusive atmosphere in academic medical centers (Fig. 4.1).

- **Organization Responsibilities**: Academic medical centers have a crucial responsibility to actively combat unconscious bias within their institutions. This includes a strong leadership commitment to setting the tone for the organization.

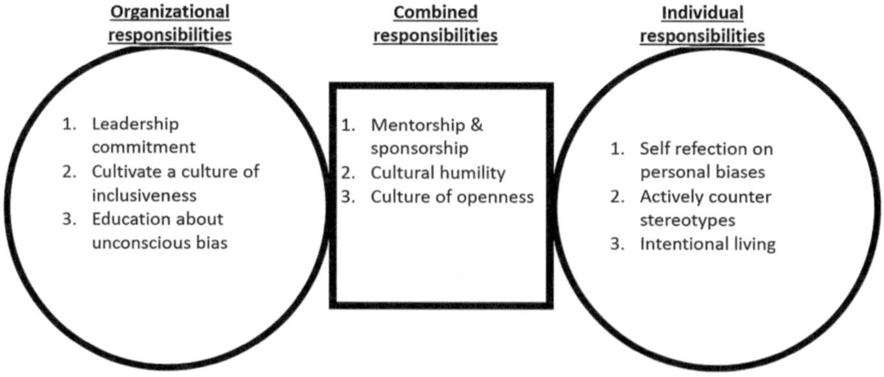

Fig. 4.1 Organizational, individual, and combined responsibilities to fight unconscious bias

Leaders should support and actively participate in creating a culture that rejects bias in all forms. This commitment is evident through developing and enforcing policies that promote diversity, equity, and inclusivity.

Leaders should also take the lead in sponsoring and participating in training sessions and workshops emphasizing the importance of diversity and the adverse effects of unconscious bias in medical settings. By leading by example, they can significantly influence the attitudes and behaviors of their staff, faculty, and students. Another important responsibility is fostering an inclusivity culture and providing ongoing education about unconscious bias. This can be achieved through mandatory educational programs for all levels of staff, including practical scenarios and role-playing exercises to help recognize and address bias in real time. Regular updates to the training content are necessary to stay current with new research and evolving understandings of bias in healthcare. Creating a safe environment for staff and patients to voice concerns about bias can lead to open dialogues and continuous improvement in addressing systemic issues.

- **Combined Responsibilities**: To effectively address unconscious bias, academic medical centers must embrace a shared responsibility that goes beyond individual actions and addresses systemic changes within their institutions. Mentorship and sponsorship are essential in this effort, providing a platform for experienced staff to guide and support others in understanding and overcoming biases. Effective mentorship involves fostering relationships where open discussions about biases and their impact on decision-making and patient care are encouraged. Similarly, sponsorship offers opportunities to underrepresented groups, ensuring they receive the same visibility and chances for advancement as their peers. Both practices help create a more equitable work environment and encourage a diverse group of future leaders.

  Cultural humility and a culture of openness are also crucial in fighting unconscious bias. This involves maintaining an open-minded approach to others' cultural identities and continuously learning and improving. Encouraging a culture of openness where employees feel at ease sharing their experiences and concerns regarding bias helps create a more inclusive atmosphere. This helps identify areas for improvement and empowers individuals to participate in the dialogue and solutions necessary to advance equity and inclusiveness across the organization. These responsibilities create a holistic approach to combating unconscious bias, promoting an inclusive atmosphere that benefits healthcare professionals and their diverse populations.
- **Practical Strategies for Physician Leaders to Fight Their Unconscious Bias at a Personal Level**: To help build physician leaders, we suggest following practical strategies for addressing unconscious bias (Fig. 4.2).
  - **Self-Reflection**: Physician leaders must dedicate time and space to reflect on their internal thoughts and biases. This allows leaders to understand better how they may affect their interactions with patients, colleagues, and staff and ultimately impact the quality of care they provide. Practicing mindfulness and reflection through journaling, meditation, or guided exercises can help leaders

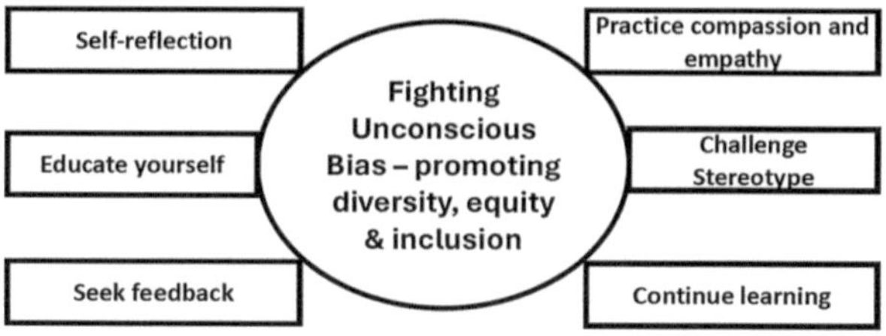

Fig. 4.2 Practical strategies for physician leaders to fight their unconscious bias at a personal level

become more self-aware and open to diverse perspectives. This journey requires humility and courage.

- **Self-Education**: Awareness of unconscious bias is crucial for physician leaders in healthcare environments. By staying up to date on the latest findings and literature, they can better understand how these biases may manifest in academic medical facilities. This understanding is essential for promoting institutional health, improving patient care, and increasing personal awareness. By recognizing and addressing unconscious bias, leaders can protect themselves and their colleagues from unfair treatment and create a more inclusive and fairer environment for staff and patients. Through ongoing education and vigilance, they can play a vital role in mitigating unconscious bias at all levels of healthcare delivery.
- **Practice Compassion and Empathy**: As physician leaders, it's essential to show compassion and empathy toward everyone in the healthcare facility, including patients, colleagues, and staff members. Leaders can create a supportive and inclusive work environment by valuing and acknowledging everyone's unique perspectives and needs. This empathetic approach promotes teamwork, boosts morale, and improves patient care and strong healthcare teams. Let's strive to listen actively, make decisions considering others' well-being, and set an example for the institution's values. Consistently demonstrating empathy and understanding helps us build a more caring and effective healthcare setting for everyone.
- **Challenge Stereotype**: Physician leaders are critical in actively challenging stereotypes and assumptions based on race, ethnicity, gender, age, or socioeconomic status. This responsibility involves consciously avoiding snap judgments that adversely affect patient care and the workplace environment. By acknowledging their implicit biases, leaders can work toward more equitable treatment and interactions within their teams and with their patients. This proactive approach supports ethical medical practices and enhances the quality of care by ensuring that all patients are seen and treated as individuals. In their daily interactions, physician leaders should strive to view each person as an individual with their own unique story and needs. This means setting aside preconceived notions and engaging with each patient and colleague with fresh eyes and an open mind. Leaders can create a sense of trust and cultivate a welcoming environment by prioritizing personalized attention and consideration. Such a practice benefits patient outcomes and contributes to a healthier, more supportive work environment that values diversity and promotes understanding among all staff.

- **Seeking Feedback**: Physician leaders should actively seek feedback from a diverse group of individuals, including peers, seniors, juniors, and patients, to overcome unconscious bias. This will help them better understand how others perceive their communication style, bedside manner, and clinical decision-making. Viewing this feedback as valuable insights that can lead to professional and personal growth rather than just criticism is essential.
- **Commit to Continue Learning**: As physician leaders, it's essential to continuously learn and be self-aware to recognize and address unconscious bias. This involves actively seeking educational resources, participating in training programs, and engaging in reflective practices. By dedicating time to this self-exploration, leaders can better understand how their biases may impact their interactions and decision-making in the healthcare setting.

Conclusion

In this chapter, we highlight the persistent issues with racism and bias in academic medicine. We address the vital role of diverse faculty in improving medical education and patient care and examine the challenges of unconscious bias and its adverse effects on professional well-being, teamwork, patient care, recruitment, and retention. We offer suggestions for organizations and individuals on self-reflection, education, empathy, challenging stereotypes, seeking feedback, and continuous learning to foster a healthcare system where belonging is a priority.

Take-Home Points

- Understanding DEI and addressing unconscious bias allows physician leaders to foster an inclusive workplace that values diverse perspectives.
- Having a better understanding of DEI and unconscious bias reduces instances of discrimination and increases job satisfaction among staff, which in turn enhances retention rates, especially among minority employees.
- Awareness and integration of DEI principles enable physician leaders to challenge the status quo and encourage more creative problem-solving.

References

1. Guevara JP, Adanga E, Avakame E, Carthon MB. Minority faculty development programs and underrepresented minority faculty representation at US medical schools. JAMA. 2013;310(21):2297–304. https://doi.org/10.1001/jama.2013.282116.
2. Butts GC, Abner P, Hess L, Palermo AS, Cotilletta B, Gianelli A, Richardson LD. Designing a road map for action to address bias and racism within a large Academic Medical Center. Acad Med. 2023;98(12):1381–9. https://doi.org/10.1097/ACM.0000000000005289.

3. Glicksman E. Unconscious bias in academic medicine: overcoming the prejudices we don't know we have. 2016. https://www.aamc.org/news/unconscious-bias-academic-medicine-overcoming-prejudices-we-don-t-know-we-have. Accessed 10 May 2024.
4. Cole KC. Ancient brains, modern dilemmas. 2012. https://www.latimes.com/opinion/la-xpm-2012-aug-12-la-oe-cole-stupidity-brain-cortex-20120812-story.html. Accessed 10 May 2024.
5. Brown B. Daring greatly: how the courage to be vulnerable transforms the way we live, love, parent, and lead. Avery; 2012.
6. Mahoney MR, Wilson E, Odom KL, Flowers L, Adler SR. Minority faculty voices on diversity in academic medicine: perspectives from one school. Acad Med. 2008;83(8):781–6. https://doi.org/10.1097/ACM.0b013e31817ec002.
7. Pololi L, Cooper LA, Carr P. Race, disadvantage and faculty experiences in academic medicine. J Gen Intern Med. 2010;25(12):1363–9. https://doi.org/10.1007/s11606-010-1478-7.
8. Price EG, Gozu A, Kern DE, Powe NR, Wand GS, Golden S, Cooper LA. The role of cultural diversity climate in recruitment, promotion, and retention of faculty in academic medicine. J Gen Intern Med. 2005;20(7):565–71. https://doi.org/10.1111/j.1525-1497.2005.0127.x.
9. Carr PL, Palepu A, Szalacha L, Caswell C, Inui T. 'Flying below the radar': a qualitative study of minority experience and management of discrimination in academic medicine. Med Educ. 2007;41(6):601–9. https://doi.org/10.1111/j.1365-2923.2007.02771.x.
10. Fang D, Moy E, Colburn L, Hurley J. Racial and ethnic disparities in faculty promotion in academic medicine. JAMA. 2000;284(9):1085–92. https://doi.org/10.1001/jama.284.9.1085.
11. Palepu A, Carr PL, Friedman RH, Ash AS, Moskowitz MA. Specialty choices, compensation, and career satisfaction of underrepresented minority faculty in academic medicine. Acad Med. 2000;75(2):157–60. https://doi.org/10.1097/00001888-200002000-00014.
12. Maxwell JC. The 17 indisputable laws of teamwork: embrace them and empower your team. HarperCollins Leadership; 2013.
13. FitzGerald C, Hurst S. Implicit bias in healthcare professionals: a systematic review. BMC Med Ethics. 2017;18(1):19. https://doi.org/10.1186/s12910-017-0179-8.
14. Center for Talent Innovation. Who perceives bias, what bias costs corporations, and how to reduce it—a new study by the Center for Talent Innovation offers answers. 2017. https://www.prnewswire.com/news-releases/who-perceives-bias-what-bias-costs-corporations-and-how-to-reduce-ita-new-study-by-the-center-for-talent-innovation-offers-answers-300486855.html. Accessed 10 May 2024.

Chapter 5
Finances in Academic Medicine

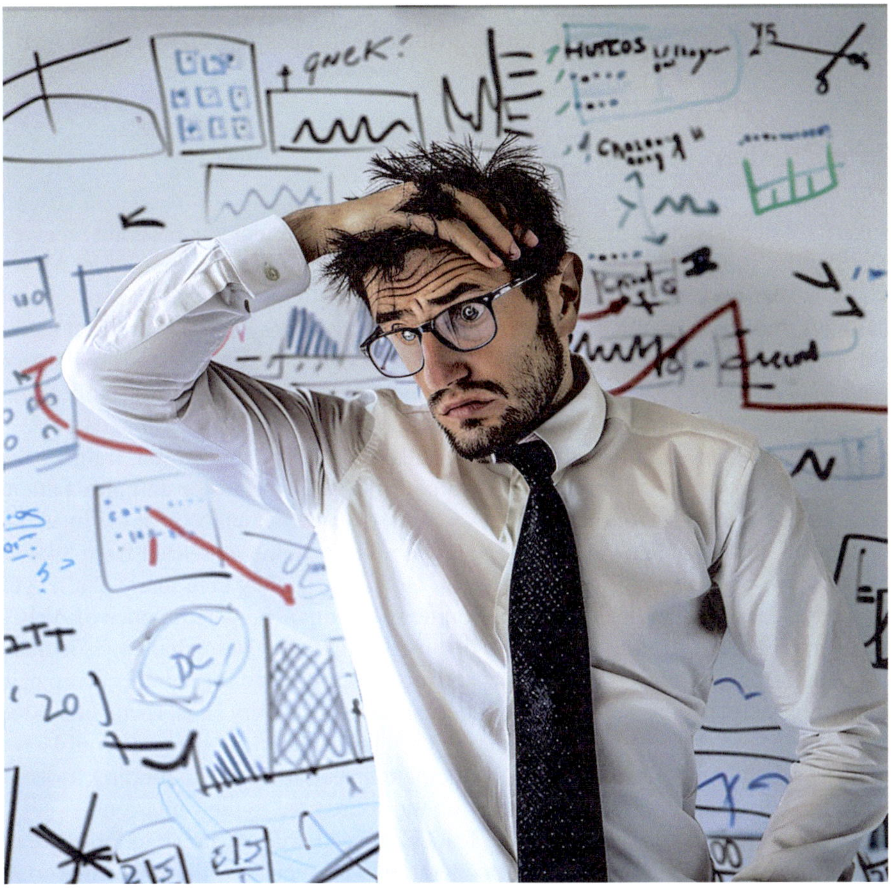

A. Djamali et al., *Emerging Leaders in Academic Medicine*,
https://doi.org/10.1007/978-3-031-80358-1_5

Case Presentation

Dr. Michaels is at the end of his training as a primary care physician and is looking forward to joining an academic medical center (AMC) in the Midwest. Dr. Michaels is interested in academic medicine because he enjoys teaching medical students and residents. He is also excited to join a group that participates in clinical research so he can be at the forefront of medicine. As he is contemplating the next steps reviewing the offer letter Dr. Michaels realizes he does not know much about finances in health care. Specifically, is his compensation fair, transparent, and competitive? Are the expectations realistic? Is there an incentive plan? And finally, how stable is the financial health of the AMC he is planning to join? Moreover, as Dr. Michaels is hoping to progress into leadership roles within his institution, and the unknowns in his own offer letter make him realize the challenges in managing finances in an AMC.

Introduction

Like Dr. Michaels, most early-stage leaders in academic medicine have not received formal education on finances in AMCs, let alone details about compensation. All we know is that doctors are supposed to make a good living after all those years of studying and training. But with the inflation, housing prices, and astronomical medical school loan repayments, early-stage physician leaders face a challenge to balance their budget. This chapter offers an opportunity for Dr. Michaels and his colleagues to make informed decisions about the financial aspects of their academic careers.

AMCs play an important role in US healthcare through innovation, training the next generation of clinicians, and providing high-quality care for complex patient populations in an educational setting. According to a recent analysis of the financial statements of 45 leading AMCs, median operating revenue increased from $4.4 to $6.9 billion (57%) from 2017 to 2022 [1]. However, as they face many challenges in today's fast-moving healthcare environment, the financial performance of AMCs measured by the operating margin has declined (Fig. 5.1). These challenges include reimbursements at a lower rate than costs, more care options for patients given new market participants, increasing use of alternative care delivery sites, rising costs due to inflation, and chronic workforce shortages [1]. This financial pressure could have severe consequences as many AMCs anticipate a need to decrease funding for education and research, even though these functions are core to their missions.

It is therefore critical for emerging leaders in academic medicine to be aware of this environment, and to participate in operational efficiency, while securing a competitive compensation packet, to enable AMCs to reinvest in their academic missions.

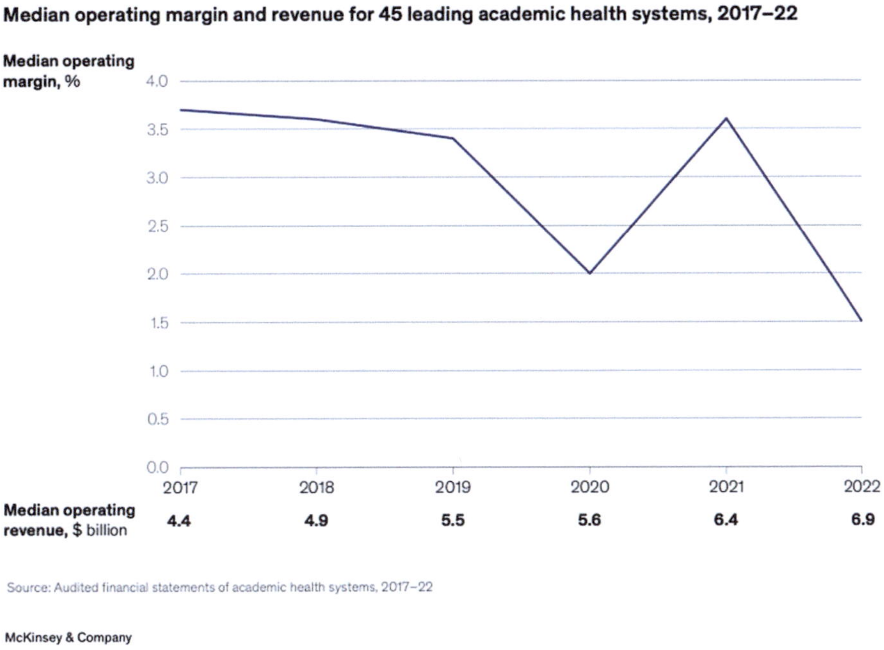

Fig. 5.1 Despite continued revenue growth, AMCs saw margins fall to 1.5% in 2022

Six Key Concepts to Understand the Operational and Financial Landscape of AMCs

Let's review six key concepts that will help physicians support their organization, while improving and monitoring their own clinical outcomes and productivity.

1. **Relative Value Units (or RVUs)**: The primary source of income for AMCs is physician billing or charges. This is where "physician productivity" contributes to operational efficiency. When a physician sees a patient, they document the visit and file charges related to the service. These charges are then sent to the insurance company or Centers for Medicare and Medicaid Services (CMS) for reimbursement. This highlights the importance of appropriate documentation and billing, so the actual physician work is captured correctly. The billing and coding department at each AMC reviews physician documentation and coding periodically to support physicians with this task. They also offer educational sessions during orientation and onboarding, to help with a better understanding of the process. In medical billing, RVUs are the weights given by the CMS under the Medicare Resource-Based Relative Value System, which was implemented for use in 1992.

   There are three types of RVUs: (1) physician work RVUs (wRVUs); (2) practice expense RVUs; and (3) professional liability insurance RVUs. The combination of all three is intended to cover the expenses of each clinical service. wRVUs are the largest component and account for the time, skill, and effort needed to deliver each specific service. With the help of wRVU, it becomes easier to compensate doctors based on their productivity.

The data for developing the original wRVUs came from a 1988 Harvard study that gathered a panel of physicians to conduct time studies and estimate the work involved in a wide variety of patient care services. Since then, CMS has updated and refined the RVU assignments—and is required by law to review them at least every 5 years, as well as when new service codes are developed. For these updates, CMS relies heavily on recommendations from the American Medical Association's Specialty Society Relative Value Scale Update Committee (RUC). There is controversy in RUC recommendations, and critics have noted that the RUC may have historically over-valued physical procedures and under-valued cognitive services. Regardless of its limitations and flaws, wRVUs tell a story of productivity and are monitored by leadership in nearly all AMCs. The 2024 Medicare Physician Fee Schedule Final Rule released by CMS in November 2023 sets the 2024 RVU conversion factor at $32.74, a decrease of $1.15, or 3.4%, from 2023. This means for every RVU generated by physicians, CMS pays $32.74. For optimal generation of RVUs, appropriate documentation and coding matters. For example, two physicians could have the exact same panel of patients and work hours, but one of them may generate higher wRVUs because of more appropriate documentation of their clinical work and optimal coding for billing.

Early-stage physician leaders should set up a meeting with their billing and coding department to learn about appropriate documentation and coding.

2. **Full-Time Equivalent (FTE)** is a metric used in healthcare to measure the number of full-time employees and part-time employees that can be translated into full-time hours. It's a way for employers to make informed decisions about finances and strategic resource allocation, especially when considering health benefits for their employees. According to the US government, an FTE is any employee who works an average of at least 30 h per week for more than 120 days in a year. Part-time employees work an average of less than 30 h per week. However, the definition of FTE may vary based on AMCs and specialties. For example, in primary care, one FTE may be defined as 32 h of direct patient contact per week, whereas 1.0 FTE acute care surgeon at a Level I center may be 24–28 service weeks per year and four to five in-house calls per month.

   It is therefore important that new physicians understand the landscape of FTEs at the organization when considering a new job.

3. **Hospital Length of Stay**: Hospital length of stay, the amount of time in an episode of hospitalization from admission to discharge, is a universal and critical metric in US healthcare. Most US hospitals have some sort of desire to reduce length of stay as well as lower hospital readmission rates. Unnecessary days in hospital may lead to increased hospital-acquired patient complications (e.g., healthcare-associated infections, falls) and increased costs for patients and healthcare systems. When the person remains in the bed following completion of

their care episode, that's when problems escalate. Imagine a patient has stabilized and is awaiting discharge and transportation to a rehabilitative care center or a skilled nursing facility. While they wait, they're still being examined by nurses whose schedules might be best spent on patients requiring more intensive help. And their chart remains within the purview of a physician whose attention can and should be spent on more at-risk individuals. While the patient stays in the bed, your labor hours aren't being maximized to their fullest extent. There's also financial incentive for moving patients to a more appropriate bed (and its attendant level of acuity). The pressing financial issue is patient throughput. The faster you can get a patient out of their high-acuity bed and onto the next level of care, the better, as that means the next patient can take their place more quickly.

   Getting patients in and out of the hospital efficiently, while delivering excellent patient-centered care, is a way to keep your revenue model rolling.

4. **Patient Experience**: Patient experience and satisfaction play crucial roles in the US healthcare system due to several key reasons. First, they directly impact health outcomes and treatment adherence. Positive patient experiences lead to better communication between patients and healthcare providers, increased trust in the healthcare system, and higher likelihood of following treatment plans, ultimately resulting in improved health outcomes and faster recovery. Second, patient satisfaction is closely tied to patient loyalty and retention. Satisfied patients are more likely to return to the same healthcare provider for future care, fostering continuity of care and long-term relationships. This not only benefits the patient by ensuring consistent and coordinated care but also helps healthcare providers build a loyal patient base and maintain financial stability. Moreover, in the current era of consumer-driven healthcare, patient satisfaction has become a key performance indicator for healthcare organizations. Positive patient experiences can enhance the reputation of healthcare facilities, attract new patients through word-of-mouth referrals and online reviews, and boost competitiveness in the healthcare market. Furthermore, patient experience and satisfaction are integral to value-based care initiatives aimed at improving quality while reducing costs. By focusing on patient-centered care and incorporating patient feedback into quality improvement efforts, healthcare providers can identify areas for enhancement, streamline processes, and deliver more personalized and effective care, thereby achieving better health outcomes at lower costs.

   Prioritizing patient experience and satisfaction in the US healthcare system is essential for improving health outcomes, fostering patient loyalty, enhancing organizational performance, and advancing the shift toward value-based care. By focusing on patient-centered care, early-stage physician leaders can not only meet the evolving needs and expectations of patients but also drive positive changes in the healthcare landscape.

5. **Care Variation**: Reducing care variation in the US healthcare system is crucial for several reasons. First, it helps ensure consistent, high-quality care for all patients, regardless of their location or provider. By standardizing best practices and treatment protocols, healthcare outcomes can be improved and unnecessary costs reduced. Second, reducing care variation promotes evidence-based medicine,

where treatments are based on scientific research and proven effectiveness rather than individual provider preferences. This leads to better patient outcomes and increased patient safety. Moreover, reducing care variation can help address health disparities by ensuring that all patients receive equitable and appropriate care, regardless of factors such as race, ethnicity, or socioeconomic status. This can contribute to reducing healthcare inequalities and improving overall population health.

By standardizing care practices, promoting evidence-based medicine, and addressing health disparities, reducing care variation is essential for improving the quality, efficiency, and equity of the US healthcare system. One of my favorite quotes addressing care variation in academic settings is "To practice evidence-based medicine, we must generate practice-based evidence." This is the value of working in AMCs, where we can change the future of medicine.

6. **Protected Time**: Protected time in academic medicine refers to dedicated periods during which faculty members can focus on research, teaching, and other scholarly activities without the distractions of clinical duties or administrative responsibilities. This time is crucial for advancing knowledge, improving patient care, and nurturing the next generation of healthcare professionals. Protected time allows researchers to delve deeply into their projects, conduct thorough experiments, analyze data, and publish their findings. This focused attention leads to high-quality research output, which contributes to the advancement of medical knowledge, development of novel treatments, and improvement of patient care outcomes. Protected time is also essential for effective teaching and mentorship. Faculty members can design innovative curricula, engage students in hands-on learning experiences, provide personalized guidance, and foster a culture of academic excellence. This not only enhances the educational experience for students but also helps cultivate a pipeline of skilled healthcare professionals who will shape the future of medicine. Furthermore, protected time enables faculty members to stay current with the latest advancements in their field, attend conferences, collaborate with peers, and participate in professional development activities. This continuous learning and networking are vital for maintaining academic rigor, fostering interdisciplinary collaborations, and enhancing the reputation of the academic institution.

It is important to note that physicians with protected time do not generate clinical revenue and are therefore unlikely to be compensated at the same rate as their peers who are fully clinical. However, this is a choice, and, after all, money is not everything! Furthermore, there is evidence that physicians with protected time have greater clinical productivity per FTE than full time clinician [2]. How can physicians request protected time? This is variable across AMCs, but in general, extramural grant funding requires non-clinical time to be assigned to a given research project. Faculty members with NIH or Foundation grants may request up to 75% protected time if they have a career development award. As we will see in the final chapter, physician scientists on tenure track may be hired with 75–80% protected time as part of their recruitment packet. Internal academic pathway mechanisms may also allow physicians to "buy-out" clinical time through innovative clinical, educational, or research projects if there is an infrastructure to support them.

Protected time in academic medicine is a precious resource that empowers faculty members to push the boundaries of knowledge, inspire the next generation of healthcare professionals, and drive innovation in patient care. Institutions that prioritize and support protected time for their faculty demonstrate a commitment to excellence, scholarship, and the advancement of healthcare for the benefit of society. Physicians with protected time should expect to earn less money than their fully clinical peers because they don't generate as much clinical revenue.

So far we have reviewed how emerging leaders in academic medicine can participate in the operational efficiency of their organization by understanding the concepts of wRVUs, FTE, hospital length of stay, patient experience, care variation, and protected time. In the next section, we will review the components of a competitive salary in modern AMCs.

Compensation Plans in Academic Medicine

Emerging leaders in academic medicine should feel comfortable asking detailed questions about their institution's compensation structure. The ideal compensation plan is transparent, equitable, standardized across the practice, and easy to understand. We should start by stating that there are as many compensation plans as there are AMCs. However, despite this wide range, there are some principles that apply to most compensation plans in academic medicine (Fig. 5.2).

- **Base Salary**: In general, base salary is what we receive in our monthly paychecks. It should consider seniority (academic rank, years since licensure), subspecialty, and expectations. For example, a full professor in neurosurgery would have a higher base salary than an assistant professor in nephrology. It is important to understand the expectations and shared consequences for failure to meet those expectations. For instance, expectations may include patient access, hours or work, relative value units or RVUs, documentation, quality, service, and citizenship. Newly hired physicians should not be surprised if they don't receive their full base salary if they don't meet the expectations.
  Regarding equitable compensation plans, most AMCs use national benchmarks for base salaries. For example, the Association of American Medical Colleges (AAMC) Annual Faculty Salary Report displays total compensation of full-time

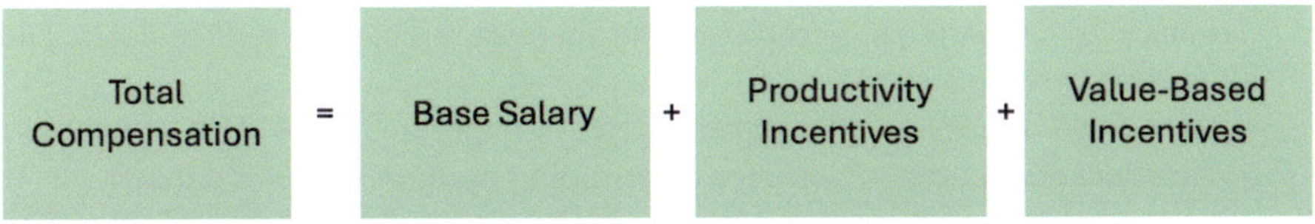

Fig. 5.2 Basic components of a compensation plan in academic medicine

medical school faculty broken out by rank, degree, department/specialty, medical school type, region, gender, and race/ethnicity. The online report is available for purchase through the AAMC Store with discounted member pricing. There are other national benchmarks, less focused on academics, which include Sullivan Cotter, Medical Group Management Association (MGMA), ECG Management Consultants, and American Medical Group Association® (AMGA). Many AMCs use a blend of compensation rates from two or more of these consulting groups or organizations.
These resources are helpful, because some of them are free to access, and provide valuable benchmarking information for early-stage physicians. For example, according to MGMA, the average salary for a physician is $377,705 per year in the United States. The highest salary for a physician in Resolve's rData is $600,000 and the lowest salary for a physician is $120,000 as of 07/30/2024.

- **Productivity Incentives**: Productivity-based incentives can play a significant role in compensation plans at AMCs. These incentives are often used to motivate and reward faculty members, physicians, and other healthcare professionals for their contributions to patient care, research, and teaching. Here are some key points for emerging physician leaders to consider:

  – Motivating Performance: Productivity-based incentives can serve as a powerful motivator for faculty members to increase their productivity and efficiency in patient care, research, and teaching activities. By linking compensation directly to performance metrics, AMCs can encourage employees to meet and exceed established goals.
  – Aligning Incentives with Organizational Goals: AMCs often have complex missions that include patient care, research, and education. Productivity-based incentives can help align individual performance with the overall goals of the institution, ensuring that employees are working toward common objectives.
  – Rewarding Excellence: By rewarding high performers with financial incentives, AMCs can recognize and retain top talent within their organizations. This can help promote a culture of excellence and continuous improvement.
  – Enhancing Recruitment and Retention: Productivity-based incentives can be used as a tool to attract and retain top talent in a competitive healthcare environment. Offering competitive compensation packages that include performance-based incentives can help AMCs attract qualified professionals and reduce turnover rates.
  – Improving Financial Performance: By tying compensation directly to productivity and performance metrics, AMCs can improve their financial performance by incentivizing employees to increase efficiency, reduce costs, and generate revenue.
  – Ensuring Fairness and Transparency: It is important for AMCs to establish clear and transparent criteria for determining productivity-based incentives to ensure fairness and equity across the organization. Employees should under-

stand how their performance is being measured and how incentives are calculated.
  - Compliance and Ethics: When implementing productivity-based incentives, AMCs must ensure that the incentive structures comply with relevant laws, regulations, and ethical standards. Incentives should not encourage inappropriate behavior or compromise patient care quality.

  Overall, productivity-based incentives can be a valuable component of compensation plans at academic medical centers, helping to drive performance, align incentives with organizational goals, reward excellence, attract and retain talent, improve financial performance, and promote fairness and transparency in compensation practices.
- **Value-Based Incentives**: Value-based incentives are another part of the variable salary. They play a crucial role in aligning the interests of clinicians with the goals of the institution, improving patient care quality, and controlling costs. Here are some key points to consider:
  - Alignment with Institutional Goals: Value-based incentives help ensure that the actions of healthcare providers align with the overall goals of the academic medical center, such as improving patient outcomes, increasing patient satisfaction, enhancing quality of care, and reducing costs.
  - Quality Improvement: By tying financial incentives to quality metrics, AMCs can motivate healthcare providers to focus on delivering high-quality care. This can lead to better patient outcomes, increased patient satisfaction, and improved overall quality of care.
  - Cost Control: Value-based incentives can also help AMCs control costs by encouraging healthcare providers to be more efficient in their use of resources. By rewarding providers for cost-effective practices, institutions can promote a culture of cost-consciousness and help reduce unnecessary expenses.
  - Physician Engagement and Retention: Incorporating value-based incentives into compensation plans can help increase physician engagement and satisfaction. When providers see a direct link between their performance and financial rewards, they are more likely to be motivated to excel in their roles and stay with the institution long term.
  - Compliance and Quality Reporting: Value-based incentives can also encourage healthcare providers to adhere to compliance standards and participate in quality reporting initiatives. By tying incentives to metrics related to compliance and quality reporting, AMCs can ensure that providers are actively working to meet regulatory requirements and continuously improve care delivery.
  - Competitive Advantage: Offering value-based incentives in compensation plans can help AMCs attract top talent in a competitive healthcare market. Physicians and other healthcare providers are increasingly looking for opportunities that offer not just competitive salaries, but also incentives tied to performance and quality outcomes.

In summary, value-based incentives in compensation plans in AMCs are essential for promoting high-quality, cost-effective care, aligning provider behavior with institutional goals, enhancing patient outcomes, and ensuring long-term success in an increasingly value-driven healthcare environment.

Assessing the Financial Health and Quality of AMCs

- **Financial Health**: Before signing a contract, early-stage physicians should examine the financial health of the organization, department, division, or practice. Financial health means stability. While a detailed analysis of hospital finances including cash flow, volume and utilization trends, labor costs, and patient revenue indicators are out of the scope of this chapter, it is acceptable to ask the employer about operating margin. A stable operating margin greater than 2% suggests relative financial security.
- Another option is to check the creditworthiness and financial trust of the AMC by looking for credit ratings issued by independent companies (available online).
  - For example, one common third-party credit rating system, Moody's, uses a letter-grade system ranging from AAA (the highest) to D (the lowest rating).
  - Fitch Ratings uses a variety of factors to assess a hospital's creditworthiness and financial health, which can then be used by investors to determine the likelihood of repayment. These factors include cash flow, operating margins, revenue defensibility, operating risk, financial profile, concentration risk, and labor market disruption. Fitch's credit rating scale for issuers and issues is expressed using the categories "AAA" to "BBB" (investment grade) and "BB" to "D" (speculative grade) with an additional +/− for AA through CCC levels indicating relative differences of probability of default or recovery for issues.
  - Similarly, Standard & Poor's (S&P) Global Ratings use a letter grade scale from AAA to D to assess a hospital's creditworthiness. The higher the grade, the lower the perceived risk. For example, a hospital with excellent financial management might receive an AAA rating, while a hospital in financial trouble might receive a D rating.
- **Quality**. The Overall Hospital Quality Star Rating (Overall Star Rating) summarizes a variety of measures across five areas of quality into a single star rating for each hospital. Once reporting thresholds are met, a hospital's Overall Star Rating is calculated using only those measures for which data are available. Hospitals report data to the Centers for Medicare & Medicaid Services (CMS) through the Hospital Inpatient Quality Reporting (IQR) Program, Hospital Outpatient Quality Reporting (OQR) Program, Hospital Readmission Reduction Program (HRRP), Hospital-Acquired Condition (HAC) Reduction Program, and Hospital Value-Based Purchasing (VBP) Program. Beginning in July 2023, Veterans Health Administration (VHA) hospitals reporting data for included

Table 5.1 Variables that are considered by CMS for Hospital Quality Ranking

Measure group	Weight used in calculation (%)
Mortality	22
Safety	22
Readmission	22
Patient experience	22
Timely and effective care	12

Table 5.2 National distribution of the Overall Star Rating based on July 2024 results (CMS)

Overall rating	Number of hospitals ($N = 4658$, %)
1 star	277 (5.9%)
2 stars	595 (12.8%)
3 stars	828 (17.8%)
4 stars	766 (16.4%)
5 stars	381 (8.2%)
N/A	1811 (38.9%)

measures are also eligible to receive an Overall Star Rating. Overall Star Ratings aren't calculated for Department of Defense (DoD) hospitals.

– **How Measure Groups Are Weighted**: For each hospital, a hospital summary score is calculated by taking the weighted average of the hospital's scores for each measure group. Table 5.1 shows the weight applied to each measure group. The hospital summary score is then used to assign star ratings to hospitals, using k-means clustering within each peer group. Note that these percentage weights are out of 100%. If a hospital has no measures in a certain measure group, the weighted percentage is redistributed proportionally to the other measure groups (Table 5.1).

CMS Hospital Quality Ratings are publicly available and may be accessed via their website. Table 5.2 shows the national distribution of the Overall Star Rating based on July 2024 results.

In summary, a good understanding of an AMC's financial and quality standings can help early-stage physician leaders in their decision making for their next job opportunity.

Final Steps: Factors to Consider Before Signing the Offer Letter

The single most important factor that will make you happy at your job is not your salary, the hospital, your colleagues, or your patients. It is your immediate boss. A supervisor who invests in you with their time, guidance, mentorship, advice, and support can make a lower salary feel like a fortune, and a dark day appear sunny. You can weather any storm with the backing of a supportive boss. The next important factors are the culture, and your peers. What is the level of trust, engagement, transparency, and burnout? And especially how friendly is the culture and work environment for your family? Finally, you need to consider neighborhood, city, and state. Once these questions have been addressed, then you can start negotiating about your salary and benefits.

Conclusion

The information provided in this chapter should equip emerging physician leaders to make an informed decision about the challenging steps of joining an AMC with a competitive salary, while contributing to patient-centered care, excellence in academics, and the financial health of the AMC.

Take-Home Points

- There is significant financial pressure in the current US Health Care System, which could have severe consequences as many AMCs anticipate a need to decrease funding for education and research, even though these functions are core to their missions.
- Emerging physician leaders can participate in the operational efficiency of their organization by understanding the concepts of wRVUs, FTE, hospital length of stay, patient experience, care variation, and protected time.
- Most compensation plans include a base salary including expectations, and a variable salary based on productivity and value-based incentives.
- Before signing a contract, emerging physician leaders should do their due diligence in understanding the financial health and quality rating of their organization.
- The most important variables for professional satisfaction of an emerging physician leader are (1) direct supervisor, (2) peers and workplace culture, (3) neighborhood, city, and state, and (4) compensation.

References

1. Levine E, Malani R, Odden A, Schulz J. Ensuring the financial sustainability of academic medical centers. Healthcare practice. McKinsey & Company; 2024.
2. Tarquinio GT, Dittus RS, Byrne DW, Kaiser A, Neilson EG. Effects of performance-based compensation and faculty track on the clinical activity, research portfolio, and teaching mission of a large academic department of medicine. Acad Med. 2003;78(7):690–701.

Chapter 6
Conflict Management, Negotiations, and the Art of Hearing and Saying No in Academic Medicine

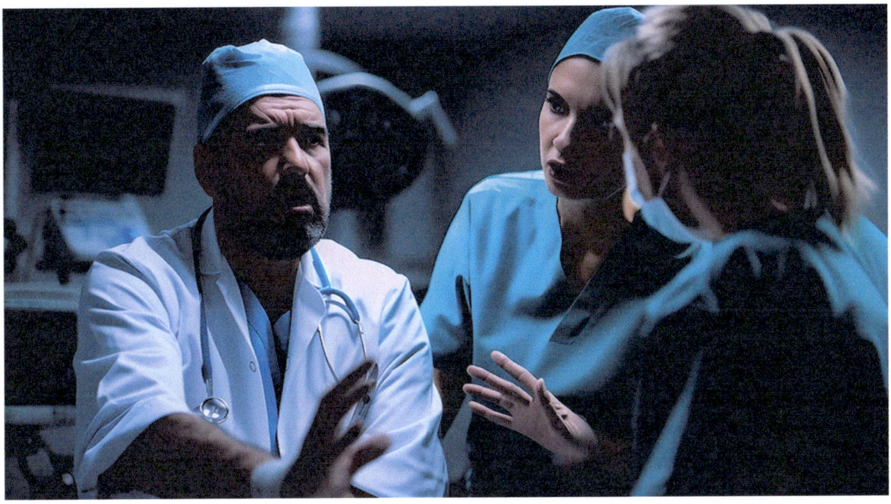

Case Presentation

A small division within an internal medicine department at an academic medical center experienced growing tensions as the priorities of one physician, Dr. Harris, were at odds with the needs of the division. Although the team had worked together smoothly for several years, a change in the finances of the institution meant they felt several changes in clinical responsibilities, research priorities, and a change in the number of trainees they were required to take on.

Dr. Harris had a strong research background and previously had a good deal of schedule flexibility to accommodate her research program. However, with the recent changes, she feels overburdened by clinical duties and that she has no time to pursue

A. Djamali et al., *Emerging Leaders in Academic Medicine*,
https://doi.org/10.1007/978-3-031-80358-1_6

her research. Other team members with higher clinical loads and more extensive experience feel undervalued and that Dr. Harris has a lack of commitment to patient care as they routinely have higher patient panels and never say anything about feeling overworked. These tensions have bubbled to the surface and led to frequent disagreements during division meetings, one-on-ones with the Division Chief, and a gossipy environment in hallways and the clinic. Meetings are unproductive and non-collaborative, junior staff are uncomfortable giving an opinion on anything, trainees have commented on the tension, and division cohesion has broken down.

Recognizing the impact this conflict was having in the division, the Division Chief met with Dr. Harris to intervene. Dr. Harris was encouraged to express her concerns openly and fully, if she allowed the Chief to do the same and present the other side of the situation. By providing a safe space for Dr. Harris to express her frustrations in full and presenting the other side in a way that emphasized shared goals all division members held, Dr. Harris was able to understand issues were stemming from differences in expectations and communication styles and not any personal conflict between "clinicians" and "researchers." Together they could work through necessary changes based on the institutional climate, Dr. Harris' strengths, and Divisional needs and create a plan to move forward. The Chief also added additional brief check-ins with Dr. Harris to ensure ongoing communication around this issue and set the expectation that other division members would be asked for their feedback on how the new plan was working.

Introduction

Conflict is an unavoidable part of our lives, and conflict management becomes even more difficult in healthcare settings where the personalities can tend toward the authoritarian and the stakes are high. Several studies have suggested that physicians tend to be perfectionists and guilt-prone, with an inflated sense of responsibility and limited emotional expressiveness [1]. Further, with increasingly demanding medical practices, physician leaders have little time to learn about conflict management. Conflicts in the academic medical institutions can lead to a toxic work environment that impacts patient care and the physician's well-being and often leading to employee turnover. In academic medical structures, young physicians often find themselves being pulled in different directions while caring for their patients. Learning about conflict management becomes crucial for us to advance in our careers.

In academic medical setups, the daily conflicts we're likely to see can vary in magnitude, such as dealing with an unhappy patient or family, working with an overburdened trainee, or working with a stressed colleague. In a survey of 5000 full-time employees in different countries, 85% of employees dealt with conflict at work to some degree, and 29% dealt with conflict frequently or constantly [2]. In another survey, 64% of respondents were experiencing a toxic personality in their current work environment, and 94% had worked with someone like that at some point in their career [3]. It is vital that physician leaders learn to manage these conflicts effectively.

Conflict Management

A conflict can be defined as a mental, emotional, or relational struggle arising from opposing demands, desires, or drives. Imagine conflict as "opposing forces." As physician leaders, we should be able to visualize the opposing forces and look at the bigger picture to get into a resolve these situations. It's important to understand that conflicts are not about winning or losing, but about understanding root causes of the conflict and negotiating solutions that are agreeable to those involved. In theory, conflicts may be an opportunity to develop self, the others, and new projects.

How to Approach to Conflict Management as Physician Leaders

After an extensive literature review, we propose a roadmap for physician leaders to use when navigating conflict management. The 5-C model of conflict management involves five principles (Fig. 6.1).

- **Step 1: Keep Calm**: Hesha Abrams, a well-known author and a master mediator, published her famous book *Hold the Calm* in 2022 [4]. In it, she explained the "hold the calm" theory: briefly, our reptilian brain arries two important small structures called the amygdala. The amygdala is in the mid-brain and is the center of fear and negativity; it controls our flight, fright, and freeze mechanisms. Activation of the amygdala causes ocular occlusion and auditory exclusion. When this happens and our visual and auditory receptors essential shutdown, we are not able to use our rational logic. This amygdala activation needs to slow down before the senses start working again. The concept of "hold the calm" is to give time to the amygdala to calm down before we respond to any kind of situation. Remember the "green circle" of emotional intelligence in Chap. 1, Fig. 1.2, and the management of your personality, emotions, biological needs, and biases? You need to be prepared for a negotiations or conflict handling meeting. Don't go to the meeting if you are hungry or tired or angry!
  Signs of Not Keeping Calm During a Conflict

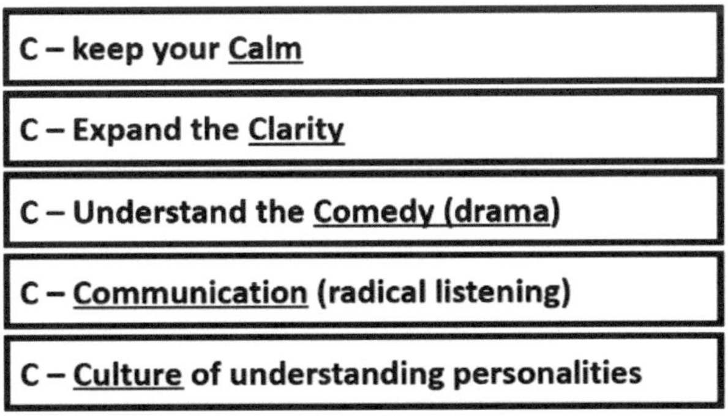

Fig. 6.1 The 5-C model of conflict management

- Defensiveness
- Panic
- Over-reaction
- Arguing

These behaviors can manifest as speaking loudly, not letting others talk, showing physical signs of anger, and many others. It is crucial that in any conflict we must analyze not only others but also ourselves, noticing whether we are keeping calm or not.

The Advantages of Keeping Calm

In times of conflict, it is crucial to understand that options are always available, and emotions need to stay down. "Keeping calm" has the following advantages:

- Regulates everyone's emotions
- Buys us time to analyze the situation
- Buys us time to come up with an appropriate response

- **Step 2: Expand Clarity**: "Clarity can change any situation." Physician leaders need to remember this critical quotation while facing a conflict. Disruptive behaviors such as bullying and raised voices confuse the leader's mind, and leaders can quickly lose focus. Wherever there is confusion, there is potential for conflict. Keeping clarity of mind and direction is essential during these situations. **Elements of Clarity**: When things are crystal clear, people around us will have less confusion, frustration, and undue stress. Clarity occurs when we have alignment and clear communication around three areas: mission, vision, and values.
  - **Mission**: The mission defines why our team comes to work every day, both individually and collectively. It provides a purpose for our daily work and acts as a north star for the team. When we understand that we all are working toward the same mission, we will try to achieve a win–win situation despite our differences. In any conflict, getting people to our central mission provides an excellent start to resolving the dispute.
  - **Vision**: The vision informs us of where we are going, what we are working toward, and how we can make a difference in the lives of others. For example, we have the vision of reaching a beautiful island while sitting in a boat. And a shark interrupts our way. The focus can quickly change from the island to the shark. Similarly, conflicts are interruptions to a beautiful destination. Keep reminding the team about the vision and direction can be extremely helpful in solving conflicts.
  - **Values**: Our values are essential behavioral expectations from all the team members. In moments of conflict, it's crucial to stick to our values, guiding us to provide space to every team member. Many disputes can be resolved just by following one's values.

Steps to Add Clarity to a Conflict: Physician leaders can use the following steps to add clarity to a conflict:

- **Situational Analysis of the Conflict**: The first step to adding clarity to conflict is to understand and describe what the problem is that's driving conflict.

This involves gathering as much information as possible and then organizing all the facts about the conflict. Sometimes, performing a simple situation analysis brings an unbiased and fresh perspective to the conflict, which can be the first step in resolving the dispute.

- **Personal Analysis**: The second step to add clarity is understanding who is involved in this conflict. Understanding the role of each person in the conflict helps physician leaders understand where the misalignment is. Further, understanding people's personalities, perspectives, and organizational positions in conflict is essential to creating a common ground for conflict resolution.
- **Future Outcome Analysis**: Physician leaders should also consider the possible outcomes of the conflict. Considering the possible outcomes helps leaders stay focused and calm during the heat of the conflict. Two essential questions to remember are: what is at risk if we cannot resolve the conflict, and what is the best outcome if we can. Sometimes making people visualize the possible outcomes and the impact of any continued conflict can cool down the heat in a conflict.
- **Self-Reflection**: During any conflict, physician leaders should do regular self-reflection to ensure that they are not part of the problem. Further, it is also essential to have periodic evaluations of the process (i.e., what has been done and what should be done next).

• **Step 3: Understand Comedy (Drama)**: Drama is common in the healthcare industry and frequently highlights the challenging aspects of human behavior. Unfortunately, drama in academic medical centers negatively impacts patient care, productivity, job satisfaction, and multidisciplinary team dynamics. Less experienced physician leaders may get caught up in the drama themselves.

The Karpman Drama Triangle: The Karpman drama triangle is a behavioral-social model of complex human interactions proposed by Dr. Stephen B. Karpman, an American psychiatrist. This triangle describes a type of destructive interaction among people during the conflict. Each position in the triangle—victim, rescuer, or persecutor—has identifiable characteristics. Let's investigate each one and discuss how it changes their position and role in a conflict (Fig. 6.2).

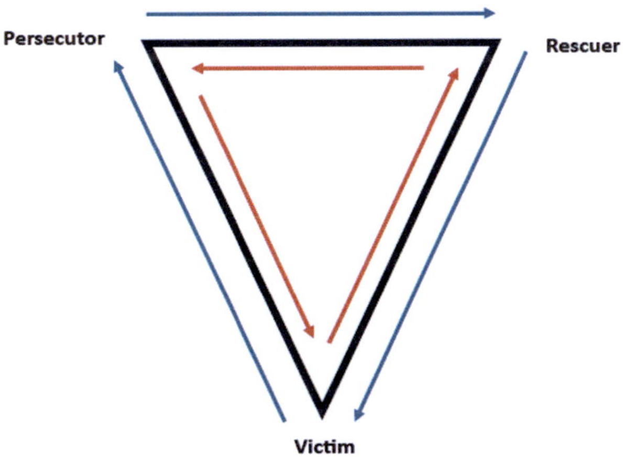

Fig. 6.2 Karpman drama triangle [5]

- **Victim (the Helpless)**: The victim in this model is not intended to represent an actual victim but rather someone feeling or acting like one. People in this role feel helpless, trapped, ashamed, and powerless. They constantly seek help to solve their problem and act as though they are dependent on others. They tend to convince themselves and others that they cannot do anything.
- **Rescuer (the Martyr)**: People playing this role gain self-esteem by "helping" others. They feel they need to fix problems and often pass off their behavior as being selfless and considerate. The rescuer feels guilty and ultimately becomes angry if they do not go to the rescue.
- **Persecutor (the Bully)**: People in this role tend to blame others for all their problems. They criticize others, act in a dominating manner, and put others down. They often act angrily and disrespectfully. They often believe that they have all the rights while others have none.

- Interestingly, all three of these roles are interchangeable. If the people in the persecutor role are blamed, they may become defensive and may switch their role to become the victim if attacked forcefully by the rescuer and/or victim, in which case the victim may also switch roles to become a persecutor. Similarly, if the people in the rescue role can't go to the rescue, they ultimately become angry and may take the role of persecutor.

How to Break the Drama Triangle? It is hard to break the drama triangle in any conflict, as people in conflict are often in denial that they are playing any part of the drama cycle. It is essential to recognize our role in the triangle in order to break it. The following steps can be taken to break the drama triangle:

- Identify and acknowledge the role we often play in the drama triangle.
- Take full responsibility for ourselves.
- Recognize the role other people are playing in the conflict.
- Dissociate ourselves from the triangle.

Sometimes even the most experienced physician leaders can find themselves pulled into the drama and conflict. Physician leaders can break the drama triangle by keeping a neutral attitude. Even if they feel defensive, they should not act from that mental state. Instead, they should use a non-reactive, non-emotional, and easy-going tone to stop the conflict.

Step 4: Communication (Radical Listening): In his famous book *The 21 Irrefutable Laws of Leadership*, John Maxwell said that "interactions fuel actions" [6]. This especially holds true in conflicts. The way we communicate is the key to whether we are going to solve the conflict or not.

In a conflict, 80% of the communication for a physician leader should be radical listening. Radical listening, also known as deep or active listening, involves fully engaging with the speaker and focusing on their words, emotions, and nonverbal cues. It requires the listener to set aside their biases and judgments and connect with the speaker to fully understand what they are trying to communicate. There's a famous saying, "wisdom is the reward you get for a lifetime of listening when you would have preferred to talk."

Principles of Radical Listening

- We are listening with our ears open.
- We understand each word.
- We understand the meaning of the words.
- We understand the meaning between the lines.
- We understand the body language of the speaker.
- We are not multitasking while listening.
- We are not interrupting.
- The speaker understands that we have the intention to listen and understand.
- We avoid expressing that the issue is not significant.
- We avoid offering unsolicited help or guidance.
- We avoid lecturing the other person.

How to Apply Radical Listening in a Conflict: Physician leaders can take the following steps to practice radical listening in a conflict:

- **Let Them Talk First**: Physician leaders should ask the people in the conflict to speak. Let them express their concerns and issues first. Always remember, "the one who listens first owns the conversation." During this step, make sure we follow the principles of radical listening. It helps us to build a space between the stimulus and the response. Also, remember we don't have to respond right after. We can always ask for more time to think through the conversation.
- **Acknowledgment**: Always acknowledge their reality. Listening and acknowledging does not mean we agree with their point, but it does make them realize that we are open to hearing all kinds of opinions.
- **Ask Questions**: If we have questions about their opinion, we should ask them. However, the questions should be genuine and focused on learning more about their views. Questions also help to make us understand the issue better. It gives them a chance to expand their thoughts on the issue and makes them see us as someone genuinely interested in learning about the issue and ultimately solving the problem.
- **Keep Our Emotions Neutral**: Even in a conflict, experienced physician leaders keep their emotions neutral. Successful leaders never let their emotions surface. Neutral feelings do not mean we agree or disagree with everything others say.
- **Our Turn**: After listening to opinions, profoundly looking into the issue, and ensuring that they seem satisfied that we are interested in solving the problem, we can say something. Before giving our opinion, always remember conflicts are not about losing or winning; instead, we need to make it a win–win scenario. Disagreements are essential to get a new perspective on the situation.

• **Step 5: Culture of Understanding the Personalities**: One of the true arts to resolving a conflict is the desire and ability to learn about the individuals involved in the conflict. As we are all different in our personalities, our way of communication, and our reactions in times of stress, physician leaders should take extra time to understand the personalities before they engage the people in the conflict.

In the previous chapter, we reviewed the characteristics of four main personality traits and considered that people may have blends of those four personalities. During a conflict, there is a tendency for personality clashes that can cause anxiety and stress in the workplace. It not only affects productivity but also creates a hostile environment. By understanding the different personalities involved in the conflict, physician leaders understand not only their personalities and preferences but also the preferences and the characters of all other people involved in the conflict. It helps us to understand the mindset of the person they are engaging with. It also helps us to consider a thoughtful, informed response.

Failure to Resolve Conflicts May Lead to a Toxic Work Environment

A toxic environment is one where negative behavior such as manipulation, bullying, and yelling are intrinsic to the organization's culture. This kind of negativity in the workplace leads to a lack of productivity and trust, is ripe for anxiety and discrimination, and leads to burnout and employee turnover.

- **Signs of a Toxic Work Environment**:
  - Communication issues: lack of communication, passive-aggressive communication, miscommunication, and unhealthy communication.
  - Cultural issues: people are mistreated, metrics matter and people don't, the environment is threatening, and micromanagement is common.
  - Behavioral issues: people bully, behave aggressively, and don't give positive feedback.
- **Impact of the Toxic Environment**:
  - Organizational failure: Toxic workplace environments erode trust and collaboration, leading to poor decision-making and undermines the goals of an organization.
  - Lack of productivity: Toxic workplaces create stress and dissatisfaction among employees, which significantly reduces their efficiency and output.
  - Actively disengaged employees: In a toxic workplace, employees often feel undervalued and unsupported, leading to disengagement and a lack of motivation to contribute positively.
  - Promotion of discrimination: Toxic workplaces often tolerate or even encourage discriminatory behaviors, creating an unfair and hostile environment that can marginalize certain groups.

Ignoring and avoiding conflict management can lead to the development of a toxic work environment. As physician leaders, we must recognize a toxic environment and promote a culture of open discussion to resolve conflicts. Physician leaders believe in the statement, "success is a daily thing." Solving everyday conflicts leads to a culture of fairness, openness, and wellness.

Thomas Kilmann Conflict Management Model [7]

While the five steps which we have described above will help you to approach conflicts in general, it is equally important to understand your natural conflict handling style. Like leadership styles, conflict management styles may be divided into five modes based on whether we are naturally assertive, or cooperative (Fig. 6.3). Each of the five modes has its own advantages and limitations. It is helpful to know your preferred Thomas Kilmann Conflict Management style (free online) so you are prepared, and try to switch styles depending on the context. It should be noted that the Thomas Kilmann Conflict Instrument is only one tool designed to help us in the difficult job of resolving conflict and managing ourselves and our fellow complex humans.

- **Competing Style**: Physicians with this style are highly assertive, with little cooperative skills. We all have a bit of competitiveness in us from our childhood years when we wanted to win a race, a soccer match, or another team sport. Physician leaders with this preferred style care more about winning the conflict than doing the right thing. They typically have a hard time to show sympathy, to listen carefully, and to compromise. But they are not afraid of conflict. They may even thrive in conflict! Let's take an example from a class of residents in training (or any group of physicians), going through a small crisis. One physician is out

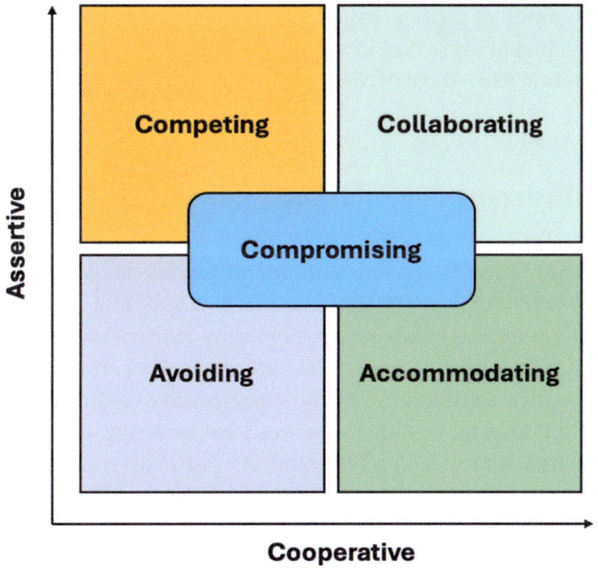

Fig. 6.3 Thomas Kilmann Conflict Management Model

sick for 3 months, and you are looking for people to step up and take a larger call load. As the leader of the practice, you send a request by email. This is an extreme example, but the person with competing style could respond immediately saying something like "When I was ill out last time, nobody stepped up to help! I am not available to take extra-call."

- **Collaborating Style**: These are physician leaders with high level of both assertiveness and cooperation. They naturally look for win–win situations. They are resourceful, think outside the box, and are willing to find opportunities to grow programs and new processes. In the example above, a physician with high collaborating style may say "This is unfortunate, but I am happy to help and take some extra-call. Let's see what everyone else is offering and develop a system to proactively address these issues in the future!"
- **Accommodating Style**: This style is highly focused on cooperation rather than assertiveness. Have you been pulled over by a policeman for a speeding ticket? Once they hand you the citation, they tell you "Thank you for your cooperation." In other words, you accommodated the process and didn't argue or complain, or... In our clinical practice example, the physician with a high accommodating style will respond immediately to the group stating "Sure, I will take extra call. Tell me how many days you need!".
- **Avoiding Style**: People with a primary avoiding style have low accommodating and competitive drives. They don't like conflict, and they don't engage in conflict. As soon as a challenging theme comes up, they either leave the conversation or change the topic. In our example, they are the last ones to respond to the email! They want to be left alone. The problem is that conflict is unavoidable.
- **Compromising Style**: This is a blended, dynamic style that may be captured with the "win some, lose some" idiom. Very helpful in healthcare, this style will allow you to concede grounds in one area and acquire new resources or opportunities in other areas. In our example, the physician leader with a high compromising style would say "Okay, I will take extra call, but I would like to have a few extra days of vacation time later in the year."

Mastering Negotiations: Essential Skills for Physician Leaders

Negotiation is a vital skill for physician leaders, especially when working with stakeholders' complex and often competing interests. As healthcare becomes increasingly collaborative, physician leaders must navigate the diverse priorities of patients, healthcare teams, administrative bodies, and external partners. This involves advocating for one's perspective and actively listening to and integrating the concerns of others, as well as fostering a collaborative environment where shared solutions can be found. As per Fisher, a trailblazer in international law and negotiation and a co-founder of the Harvard Negotiation project, "Negotiation is not about defeating your opponent. Negotiation is about creating an agreement where both sides can succeed" [8].

The Foundation of Negotiation

Negotiations are rarely just one-time events, but rather they are an ongoing process. The aim is to reach a win–win agreement, and this can be achieved when both parties must set reasonable goals while remaining open to flexibility throughout the bargaining. Whether negotiating with hospital administration, department leadership, junior colleagues, or nursing staff, physician leaders must steer negotiations toward mutually beneficial solutions. This approach fosters collaboration and ensures all parties feel valued and heard, ultimately leading to more sustainable and positive outcomes. In his book "Bargaining for Advantage," Richard Shell presents a strategy of information-driven bargaining focusing on six essential elements crucial for successful negotiation [9]. This approach emphasizes the significance of thorough preparation, attentive listening, and emotional intelligence from all parties involved. By entering negotiations with clear objectives, physician leaders can significantly benefit from implementing this strategy. The upcoming section will explore these six critical elements from "Bargaining for Advantage" and demonstrate how physician leaders can incorporate them into daily routines (Fig. 6.4).

First Foundation: Development of Personal Bargaining Style

Determining your conflict threshold and attitude is essential for developing one's bargaining style. Shell stresses the importance of understanding one's negotiation style, with flexibility critical to success: it's crucial to balance assertiveness with consideration for others [9] (Fig. 6.5). Physician leaders must always negotiate to establish successful future relationships, using a problem-solving or compromise-focused approach. For example, a physician leader negotiating work hours with a practice may aim for fewer night shifts but should remain flexible flexibility to meet the practice's needs while taking care of their well-being. Finding a balance between assertiveness and empathy nurtures long-term relationships. While immediate gains may seem appealing, they could give the impression that one is not a team player.

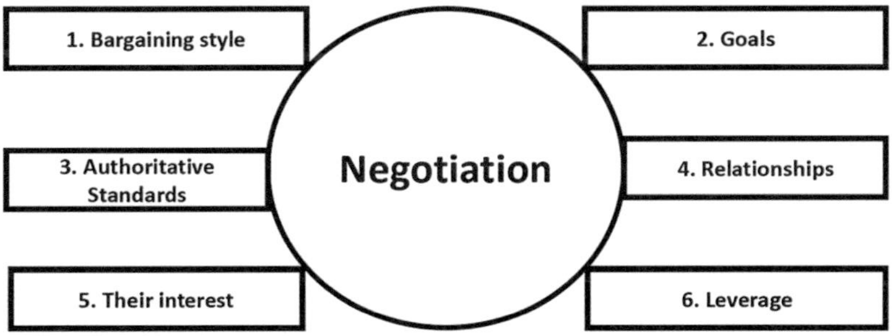

Fig. 6.4 Foundations of effective negotiation. (Concept adopted from "Bargaining for Advantage" [9])

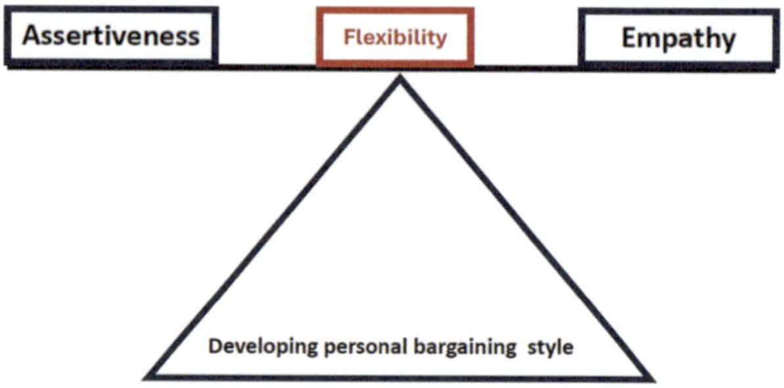

Fig. 6.5 The bargaining style should balance assertiveness and empathy

On the other hand, being willing to compromise in the short term can lead to significant benefits in the future as one builds a good reputation and rapport. Achieving this delicate equilibrium assists physician leaders in enhancing their influence with others. As a renowned leadership coach, John Maxwell aptly says, "Leadership is all about influence, nothing less, nothing more" [10]. As it relates to the patient–physician relationship, this approach is a critical part of shared decision-making. This collaborative process between physician and patient helps ensure the best decisions are made. Shared decision-making is vital for patient-centered care as it strengthens the bond by openly sharing expertise. Making medical choices is easier when patients are fully informed and involved. Patients are more likely to accept decisions they are involved in, enhancing the meaningful human experience of the patient–physician relationship based on trust and mutual respect. For example, a physician discussing treatment plans with a patient might explain various options and consider the patient's lifestyle and preferences, leading to a mutually agreed-upon plan [11].

Second Foundation: Setting Realistic Goals

Setting practical and achievable goals is crucial whenever entering negotiations, particularly in healthcare leadership. This strategic approach ensures that negotiations are focused and effective, increasing the chances of a successful result. Identify which parts of the agreement are up for negotiation, such as salary, work hours, duties, perks, and other terms. Knowing these aspects allows for a more adaptable negotiation plan. Once you've identified the negotiable points, prioritize them according to their significance to the overall objectives. For example, some may prioritize work–life balance, while others may value salary or career growth opportunities more. Prioritizing helps concentrate efforts where they are most important. It's equally crucial to determine what is non-negotiable. These requirements must be fulfilled for the agreement to move forward. By having this list, leaders can ensure that essential needs are not overlooked, preserving the deal's integrity. As Shell stated, "Know what you want, why you want it, and what you are willing to sacrifice to achieve it" [9]. This concept emphasizes the significance of being self-aware and transparent in negotiations. Knowing one's own motivations and boundaries enables one to employ more strategic and successful negotiation strategies. Documenting these items ensures that all aspects are considered, and nothing is overlooked during negotiations. It serves as a reference point to maintain focus and direction. Both parties in the negotiation should come well prepared with a list of negotiable aspects of the deal. Preparation includes understanding the other party's needs and constraints, which can foster a more collaborative and mutually beneficial negotiation process.

Third Foundation: Determination of the Authoritative Standards

In the third foundation, it's essential to establish clear negotiation standards, for which thorough planning is crucial. Each negotiator should have defined goals and share supporting data, as both sides should be able to justify their requests. Preparation should anticipate counterarguments and plan responses, providing an early advantage for future negotiations. As an example, in medical practice, it is easy to find standard salary benchmarks for various specialties nationwide when entering into a contract negotiation. These benchmarks serve as a baseline, acknowledging each physician's and practice's individuality. Negotiations may be affected by multiple factors like qualifications, experience, demand, and patient demographics, resulting in salaries falling at different points within the range. This adaptability enables individuals to distinguish themselves, proving advantageous for employers and employees. An organization helping doctors gain patients might propose a lower salary initially, citing their support as a significant benefit. This support can include marketing assistance, patient referrals, or administrative help, which can be highly valuable for new or transitioning physicians. Conversely, physicians with extensive experience, special training, research contributions, or unique skills may have substantial grounds to negotiate for a higher salary. Their added value to the practice can justify a higher compensation package. Setting clear standards for negotiation, defining goals, exchanging supporting data, and preparing for opposing arguments are essential. These practices ensure that negotiations are grounded, focused, and beneficial for both parties.

Fourth Foundation: Focusing on Relationships

The fourth foundation centers on establishing reciprocity norms and prioritizing relationship building. Engaging with personnel across different sectors enhances credibility and grants access to specific resources. By offering small compromises, demonstrating goodwill, and making personal contributions, leaders can establish a strong foundation for enduring relationships that result in mutual advantages. According to Simon Sinek, a British American author and motivational speaker in the field of business leadership, "Leadership is not about being in charge. It's about taking care of those in your charge" [12]. Although nearly 40 years on, renowned leadership expert Ken Blanchard's maxim "The key to successful leadership today is influence, not authority" is as applicable now as when he first said it [13]. This principle can be seen in medical settings through the dynamic between physician leaders and trainees. Trainees gain more responsibilities, chances to learn, and independence in exchange for helping with patient care and the guidance they receive during training. In employer–employee relationships, physicians should be mindful of reciprocity challenges that could create trust too quickly or lead to feelings of obligation. While striving for mutual advantage, both sides should acknowledge the professional aspect of negotiations, upholding trustworthiness and mutual respect as core values.

Fifth Foundation: Exploration of Other Individual Interests

In the fifth foundation, exploring each party's interests is essential. Identifying what each party values and the decision-makers involved is crucial. Like the discovery phase in legal proceedings, understanding the other party's priorities is vital. Physician leaders should collaborate with others to align their actions with mutual interests, turning negotiations into a joint effort toward shared goals. Understanding each party's priorities, such as financial contributions, scholarly impact, and academic reputation, is essential for successful negotiations. By contributing to each other's objectives, both sides can create value and pursue additional goals.

Sixth Foundation: Establishment of Leverage

The sixth key to successful negotiation is building leverage. In the medical realm, this can involve having unique technical skills, industry connections, or reliability in handling tasks others avoid. This can make a physician leader invaluable and boost patient referrals and procedure volumes. While leverage is essential, it should be paired with cooperation and compromises for the best results for everyone involved. Just as in furniture assembly or construction when too much leverage and pressure can combine for disastrous results, so too can over-leveraging a skill or unique asset in workplace negotiation. Physician leaders must have a solid grasp of these six foundations. By mastering these principles, they can effectively handle conflicts and positively impact patient care outcomes, team dynamics, and overall organizational success.

Applying "The Four Steps of the Walk in the Woods" Concept to Physician Leadership

Marcus and colleagues presented the idea of "The Walk in the Woods," offering a detailed approach to promoting interest-based negotiation and conflict resolution [14, 15]. Let's explore how physician leaders can utilize this concept to effectively navigate daily conflicts and negotiations. Physician leaders can boost their skills in

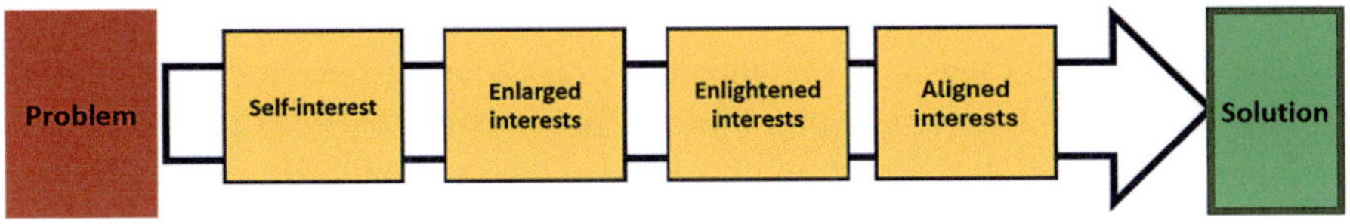

Fig. 6.6 Application of Walk in Woods for physician leaders. (Concept adopted from "The Walk in the Woods: A Step-by-Step Method for Facilitating Interest-Based Negotiation and Conflict Resolution") [14]

tackling complex healthcare issues promoting collaboration and innovation by using "The Four Steps of the Walk in the Woods" framework (Fig. 6.6).

Step 1: Self-Interests: Physician leaders must clearly articulate their priorities and concerns while also actively listening to the perspectives of others within their teams and across stakeholders. This step ensures that personal agendas align with broader organizational goals, distinguishing genuine self-interest from purely selfish motives. By openly communicating and validating diverse viewpoints, leaders promote a culture of transparency and mutual respect essential for effective teamwork and decision-making in healthcare settings.

Step 2: Enlarged interests: Physician leaders must be open to and facilitate discussions identifying common ground and reframing issues to stimulate creative problem-solving. Leaders can leverage this multi-dimensional understanding to comprehensively devise innovative solutions that address complex healthcare challenges by fostering an environment where diverse perspectives are valued.

Step 3: Enlightened Interests: Physician leaders should encourage brainstorming sessions to explore potential solutions for the problems. They prioritize strategies that promise mutual benefits and alignment with organizational values and patient care goals. Engaging stakeholders in evaluating and refining these options ensures that proposed solutions are innovative but also practical and sustainable within the healthcare environment.

Step 4: Aligned Interests: Physician leaders should negotiate with a focus on creating outcomes where all parties involved perceive significant benefits—a "win–win" scenario. They secure commitments to agreed-upon solutions and develop detailed implementation plans with clear accountability measures. Leaders foster a culture of collaboration and commitment that drives positive change and enhances healthcare delivery outcomes by cultivating consensus and ensuring buy-in from all stakeholders.

By following "The Four Steps of the Walk in the Woods," physician leaders can have a structured method for making decisions, negotiating, and leading in healthcare. By aligning personal goals with organizational aims, promoting teamwork, and seeking solutions that benefit everyone involved, leaders can successfully navigate challenges and guide their teams toward sustainable enhancements in patient care and organizational achievements.

In summary, mastering negotiation is vital for physician leaders as it helps them manage the different needs of stakeholders while keeping patient care as the top priority. Physician leaders can promote a collaborative atmosphere by creating a personal negotiation style that combines assertiveness with empathy, setting achievable goals, maintaining high standards, prioritizing relationship building, understanding the interests of all parties, and utilizing their strengths. This method tackles current issues and cultivates lasting partnerships and practical solutions, leading to improved patient results and organizational achievements.

Once again, there are no good or bad styles in negotiations or conflict handling. In fact, many people have blended styles. But recognizing these different modes allows you to navigate through the conflict or negotiations with more flexibility.

The Art of Hearing and Saying "No"

A common situation that will bring all these skills and competencies together is when you receive, or must tell someone else, no. It is a critical life skill that contributes to personal growth, professional development, and agile thinking, and can create healthier relationships with others [16].

- Resilience Building: Rejection is a part of life, and handling it appropriately helps build resilience, allowing us to bounce back from setbacks. Facing rejection triggers emotions, but it also provides an opportunity to process and manage those feelings. Connecting with others—friends, family, or mentors—enhances resilience by offering support and understanding. Each "no" can be a stepping-stone toward personal growth, reinforcing that resilience is about thriving despite adversity.
- Growth and Learning: Hearing "no" offers valuable feedback and learning opportunities, allowing reflection on what's important and what can be improved. Handling rejection is essential in life, and resilience grows when we effectively cope with it. While rejection can feel like defeat, it can also be a powerful motivator. Understanding why you received a "no" guides your learning and opens new directions, showing that resilience and growth often emerge from facing rejection head-on.
- Improved Negotiating Skills: Understanding and accepting "no" can enhance your negotiating skills by helping you recognize boundaries and find mutually beneficial solutions. Rejection teaches you to manage emotions and stay focused during negotiations. It encourages active listening and understanding the other party's perspective, building empathy and trust. Each rejection is an opportunity to refine your strategies and become more flexible, turning "no" into a chance to grow and improve your negotiation skills.
- Emotional Maturity: Learning to accept "no" gracefully demonstrates emotional maturity, showing you can handle disappointment without taking it personally or reacting negatively. Emotionally mature individuals empathize with others, treat-

ing them with respect and expecting the same in return. They recognize and manage their emotions healthily, preventing inappropriate reactions. Being adaptable and open-minded enhances their ability to compromise and find solutions. Setting boundaries without guilt and respecting others' boundaries foster healthy interactions, making each "no" an opportunity for growth and emotional development [17].

- Better Relationships: Accepting "no" can improve both personal and professional relationships by showing respect for others' decisions and boundaries, fostering mutual respect and trust. Saying no establishes healthy boundaries, maintaining individuality and preventing resentment. It encourages understanding and mutual respect, strengthening the relationship. Setting boundaries nurtures self-empowerment and authenticity, promoting a stronger connection by honoring your well-being.
- Enhanced Problem Solving: Facing "no" forces you to think creatively and explore alternative paths, leading to innovative solutions. Rejection enhances problem-solving abilities by cultivating flexibility and creativity. Understanding why you received a "no" requires empathy, helping you see situations from different angles and leading to comprehensive solutions. Each "no" builds resilience, teaching you to persist, explore alternatives, and find innovative ways to overcome challenges, turning rejection into a learning opportunity that sharpens your problem-solving skills.

Conclusions

Workplace conflicts can have a negative impact if we see a conflict as something to avoid or be afraid of. However, if we embrace the concept that conflicts are a normal part of being human and learn to deal with them, we will approach conflicts with more confidence and compassion. Handling conflicts well leads to an improved understanding of the tasks, team development, and quality of group decision-making.

Take-Home Points

- Conflicts happen daily, and physician leaders need to consider conflicts as a new opportunity.
- When in conflict, apply the 5-C model to handle the dispute:
  - Keep the Calm
  - Expand the Clarity
  - Understand Comedy (drama)
  - Communication (Radical listening)
  - Develop a Culture of understanding personalities.

- Failure to resolve conflicts leads to a toxic work environment.
- It's the job of physician leaders to recognize a toxic work environment and take every step to resolve disputes.
- Physician leaders must navigate diverse stakeholder priorities to keep their goals central.
- Effective negotiation can be a contentious process requiring flexibility and realistic goal setting for win–win outcomes.
- Success in negotiation involves a balanced bargaining style, clear goals, authoritative standards, and strong relationship building.

References

1. Thomas M, Bigatti S. Perfectionism, impostor phenomenon, and mental health in medicine: a literature review. Int J Med Educ. 2020;11:201–13. https://doi.org/10.5116/ijme.5f54.c8f8.
2. Overton AR, Lowry AC. Conflict management: difficult conversations with difficult people. Clin Colon Rectal Surg. 2013;26(4):259–64. https://doi.org/10.1055/s-0033-1356728.
3. Kusy M, Holloway E. Toxic workplace! San Francisco: Jossey-Bass; 2009.
4. Abrams H. Holding the calm: the secret to resolving conflict and defusing tension. Berrett-Koehler Publishers; 2020.
5. The Drama Triangle Explained. https://leadershiptribe.com/blog/the-drama-triangle-explained#:~:text=The%20Drama%20Triangle%20was%20first,and%20ineffective%20response%20to%20conflict. Accessed 6 Dec 2023.
6. Maxwell JC. The 21 irrefutable laws of leadership: follow them and people will follow. HarperCollins Leadership; 2022.
7. Kilmann R. Mastering the Thomas-Kilmann conflict mode instrument. Kilmann Diagnostics; 2023.
8. Fisher R, Ury WL, Patton B. Getting to yes: negotiating agreement without giving in. 3rd ed. Penguin Books; 2011.
9. Shell R. Bargaining for advantage: negotiation strategies for reasonable people. Gildan Media, LLC; 2014.
10. Maxwell JC. Becoming a person of influence: how to positively impact the lives of others. HarperCollins Leadership; 2006.
11. Aziz F. The power of shared decision-making in medical settings. WMJ. 2023;122(1):5–6. https://www.ncbi.nlm.nih.gov/pubmed/36940111.
12. Sinek S. Leaders eat last: why some teams pull together and others don't. Portfolio. 2017.
13. Blanchard K, Zigarmi P, Zigarmi D. Leadership and the one minute manager: increasing effectiveness through situational leadership. William Morrow; 1985.
14. Marcus LJ, Dorn BC, McNulty EJ. The walk in the woods: a step-by-step method for facilitating interest-based negotiation and conflict resolution. Negot J. 2012;28:337–49.
15. Marcus LJ, McNulty EJ, Henderson JM, Dorn BC. You're it: crisis, change, and how to lead when it matters most. PublicAffairs; 2021.
16. Lench HC, et al. Exploring the toolkit of emotion: what do sadness and anger do for us? Soc Personal Psychol Compass. 2016;10(1):11–25. https://doi.org/10.1111/spc3.12229.
17. Rowe AD, Fitness J. Understanding the role of negative emotions in adult learning and achievement: a social functional perspective. Behav Sci (Basel). 2018;8(2):27. https://doi.org/10.3390/bs8020027. PMID: 29461487; PMCID: PMC5836010.

Chapter 7
Creating a Culture of Engagement and Combating Burnout

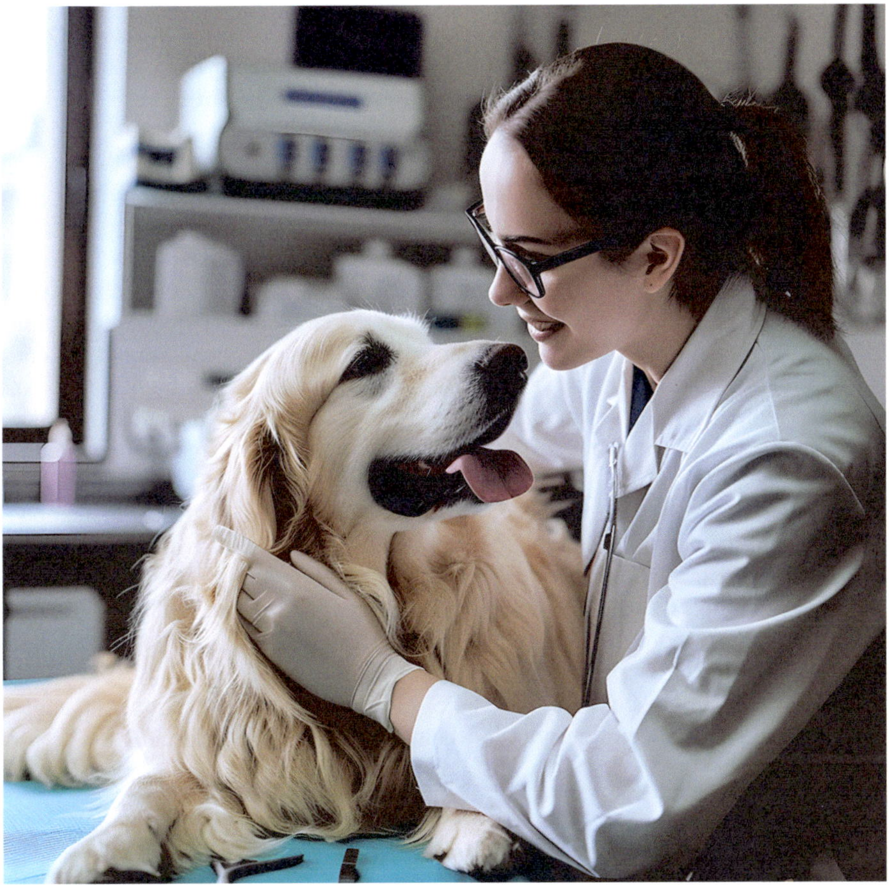

A. Djamali et al., *Emerging Leaders in Academic Medicine*,
https://doi.org/10.1007/978-3-031-80358-1_7

Case Presentation

Dr. Mohamed, the latest addition to the institution's cardiology department, has recently finished her rigorous training and is excited to start her new position. Even though she dealt with numerous obstacles and stresses during her training, she now races the reality of managing clinical duties, administrative work, team conflicts, and maintaining a work–life balance day in and day out. Unfortunately, her initial enthusiasm has waned as she feels drained and frustrated, indicating signs of burnout.

As a young physician leader, Dr. Mohamed recognizes the importance of engagement and avoiding burnout for her career success, personal well-being, and the health of her team and organization. In general, engaged leaders are more productive, have stronger communication skills, and are excellent team motivators. On the other hand, burnout can result in less productivity, increased cynicism, and a sense of helplessness, which can further worsen physician leaders' stress.

Introduction

Burnout can significantly influence an individual's overall health, resulting in fatigue, sleep problems, stress, and sadness. Dr. Mohamed may find it challenging to focus and make sound decisions, which could affect her patients' quality of care. Burnout can negatively impact a health organization, leading to higher employee turnover, more absences, lower patient satisfaction, and increased medical mistakes. Physician leaders must recognize the signs of burnout and take steps to prevent it for them and their teams.

To foster effective leadership and organizational health, it is critical to acknowledge the significance of managing engagement and burnout. Institutions can help new leaders like Dr. Mohamed to properly carry out their jobs by recognizing warning signs and implementing methods to handle stress and foster involvement. In the end, this support improves their well-being and benefits the larger healthcare environment in which they operate.

This chapter will discuss the importance of physician leaders creating an engaging environment to prevent burnout for themselves and their teams.

Creating an Environment of Engagement

Whether in clinical settings, research responsibilities, or administrative roles, physician leaders work in varied teams in various settings in academic centers. In the clinical realm, they work with colleagues, physician assistants, nurses, and trainees at multiple levels. In addition to coordinating treatment, physician leaders must ensure that everyone in the team knows their duties. This cooperation is essential to delivering excellent patient care and preserving a productive and encouraging work atmosphere. A good clinical team must have mutual respect, effective communication, and shared goals. In research settings, physician leaders often guide multidisciplinary teams, including researchers, laboratory technicians, and data analysts. They must foster an environment encouraging innovation, critical thinking, and rigorous scientific inquiry. This involves overseeing the research process, mentoring junior researchers, and ensuring compliance with ethical standards and regulatory requirements.

Administrative tasks further complicate their responsibilities. In addition to developing and implementing policies, physician leaders must handle resources and negotiate the complexities of healthcare administration. This calls for a strategic vision, the capacity for complex decision-making, and the ability to balance conflicting needs and priorities. Like so many things in leadership, engagement is not an all or nothing proposition; engagement in the workplace exists on a continuum. Gallup breaks down engagement into three broad definitions (Table 7.1) and includes definitions of what employee behavior looks like in each category and the result that behavior has on a workplace. For 2023, Gallup reports that 23% of the US workforce identified as Engaged, 16% as Actively Disengaged, and the majority of 61% identifying as Not Engaged. Definitions of each and the effect of each category on the workplace are outlined in Table 7.1.

Emotional intelligence, robust leadership abilities, and clinical knowledge are crucial for effectively managing employee engagement in the diverse roles physician leaders occupy. As renowned American leadership coach John Maxwell famously stated, “Everything rises and falls on leadership” [1]. For physician leaders, establishing influence with each team member is more vital than concentrating solely on their duties. John Maxwell further emphasized, “Leadership is all about influence, nothing less, nothing more” [2].

Leadership Characteristics That Lead to an Environment of Engagement

By adopting the following essential characteristics, physician leaders can increase their influence on the team members and generate an environment of engagement.

Table 7.1 Characteristics of different levels of engagement at the workplace

Category	Definition	Result
Engaged	Employees who are involved in, enthusiastic about, and committed to their work and workplace	Employees drive performance, innovation, and move the organization forward
Not engaged	Employees are psychologically unattached to their work and company	Employees put time, but not energy or passion, into their work
Actively disengaged	Employees aren’t just unhappy at work, they are resentful that their needs are not being met	Employees act out on their unhappiness and create toxic workplaces

1. **Value People**: Recognizing and appreciating team members' hard work and dedication is essential for fostering a motivated and committed team. Simple acts like offering praise in meetings or sending personalized notes of gratitude can significantly increase morale. Consistently acknowledging individual and team achievements helps create a culture of appreciation and respect. As Peter Drucker wisely stated, "The most important thing in communication is hearing what isn't said," underlining the importance of recognizing team members' unspoken efforts and contributions [3]. By actively valuing and appreciating these contributions, physician leaders can build trust, promote positive behaviors, and enhance team cohesion and performance.

   Offering helpful feedback is vital to showing appreciation for others, enabling them to develop and reach their objectives. Feedback must be clear, actionable, and given in a supportive way, focusing on actions rather than personal traits [4]. This strategy ensures that feedback is well received and leads to significant improvements. American football Coach John Wooden emphasized the significance of this approach, stating "A coach is someone who can give correction without causing resentment" [5]. Physician leaders can support team members in identifying areas for growth, improving their abilities, and realizing their full potential. This benefits both the individual and the team, contributing to overall success. Recognizing and celebrating successes, whether individual accomplishments or team milestones, are crucial for reinforcing positive behaviors and lifting spirits. By acknowledging achievements, physician leaders can motivate their team members, showing that their efforts are respected and valued. This fosters a culture of excellence and ongoing enhancement. Remember the wise words of leadership coach Dale Carnegie, "People may work for a paycheck, but they go the extra mile for recognition, praise, and rewards" [6].

   Creating a warm and inclusive atmosphere where each team member feels appreciated and respected is essential for fostering a sense of belonging. When team members feel valued, they are more likely to be engaged, committed, and motivated. This sense of belonging can be cultivated through clear communication, active listening, and a genuine embrace of diverse perspectives. Maya Angelou, a renowned poet and civil rights advocate, eloquently captured this sentiment with her words, "People will forget what you said, people will forget what you did, but people will never forget how you made them feel" [7]. By promoting a supportive and diverse environment, physician leaders can ensure that every team member feels respected and valued, enhancing teamwork, job satisfaction, and overall team achievements.
2. **Help People Grow**: Investing in the professional development of team members is crucial for fostering an energetic team environment. Supporting their career aspirations and encouraging them to pursue further certifications or education demonstrates leaders' commitment to their team's future achievements. This emphasis on professional growth enhances individual competencies and prepares the team to tackle new challenges and adapt to the evolving demands of the healthcare industry.

Mentorship plays a vital role in guiding individuals forward. Effective mentorship from leaders encourages sharing knowledge, improving skills, and offering career advice. Mentors provide valuable insights, draw from their experiences, and give helpful feedback to help mentees navigate their career paths successfully. A continuous improvement and innovation culture is fostered by supporting team members' professional growth through mentorship. As individuals progress, they become more motivated, engaged, and committed to contributing to the team's success. This holistic approach to professional development helps ensure the team stays skilled, confident, and capable of achieving its goals.

3. **Enhance Open Communication**: Promoting transparent and open communication within the team is crucial for establishing a cohesive and productive working environment. Allowing team members to freely share their ideas, concerns, and feedback fosters trust and collaboration. Open communication facilitates the smooth exchange of information, essential for resolving conflicts and making well-informed decisions. Remembering Stephen Covey's advice, "Seek first to understand, then to be understood," emphasizes the importance of listening and understanding others before sharing your thoughts [8]. Prioritizing open communication ensures that every team member is respected and acknowledged, enhancing teamwork and effective problem-solving.

   Effective communication is critical to team alignment and success. When everyone is well informed and working toward common goals, misunderstandings are minimized, and productivity is maximized. By actively listening and being perceptive, leaders can create an environment where team members collaborate efficiently and support each other effectively. This fosters a culture of engagement and commitment, achieving the best outcomes.
4. **Lead by Example**: Demonstrating the behaviors and attitudes you wish to see in your team is essential for effective leadership. Leading by example sets a clear standard for others to follow and inspires them to reflect positive traits such as integrity, dedication, and professionalism. When leaders exhibit the values and strong work ethic they expect from their team, it reinforces those behaviors and cultivates a culture of accountability and excellence. Renowned leadership expert John C. Maxwell emphasizes, "A leader is one who knows the way, goes the way, and shows the way," emphasizing the importance of leaders as role models who guide their team through actions and words [9].

   Leaders who embody the qualities they seek in their team can build trust and credibility. Team members are more likely to respect and follow a leader who shows consistency between their words and actions. This alignment fosters reliability and predictability, crucial for maintaining a stable and cohesive team environment. Mahatma Gandhi's quote, "Be the change you wish to see in the world," emphasizes the power of personal example in driving change and influencing others [10]. By consistently exhibiting desired behaviors, leaders create a positive influence that motivates and inspires their team to strive for excellence.
5. **Build Strong Relationships**: Building strong and respectful relationships is essential for effective leadership and team unity. Knowing each team member's

strengths, weaknesses, and motivations enables physician leaders to provide tailored support that fosters individual growth and team dynamics. Connecting with the team personally and professionally helps build trust and demonstrates genuine care for their well-being and success. Remember Dale Carnegie's words, "You can make more friends in two months by showing interest in others than you can in two years by trying to get others interested in you" [6]. This quote highlights the significance of showing authentic interest and empathy toward the team to create meaningful connections. Cultivating strong relationships creates a supportive atmosphere where team members feel valued and understood. When team members feel respected and acknowledged, they become more engaged, motivated, and committed. This sense of belonging and mutual respect enhances teamwork and communication, leading to a more efficient and united team. John C. Maxwell's quote, "People don't care how much you know until they know how much you care," emphasizes the importance of empathy and personal connections in leadership [11]. By nurturing strong relationships, leaders can establish a positive work environment that encourages team members to give their best, knowing their efforts are valued and respected.

6. **Empower Others**: Encouraging team members to take ownership of their work and empowering them to make decisions can boost their confidence and sense of responsibility. Trusting others with important tasks and decision-making authority can increase job satisfaction and motivation. When team members feel valued and trusted, they are more likely to take initiative, think creatively, and offer innovative solutions. Theodore Roosevelt once said, "The best executive is the one who has sense enough to pick good men to do what he wants done, and self-restraint enough to keep from meddling with them while they do it" [12]. This quote emphasizes the importance of choosing capable individuals and allowing them the freedom to excel in their roles without unnecessary interference.

   Empowering team members not only boosts their dedication to the team's goals but also contributes to the overall success. When individuals are given the chance to take charge of their work, they form a deeper connection to the results and become more committed to achieving the team's objectives. This feeling of ownership increases engagement and responsibility, prompting team members to exceed expectations to ensure project success. Additionally, empowerment fosters a culture of continuous growth and learning, motivating team members to seek new knowledge and skills to improve their performance actively. As leadership expert John C. Maxwell famously said, "Leaders are great not because of their authority, but because of their ability to empower others" [9]. By creating an environment where team members are empowered, leaders can cultivate a more dynamic, innovative, and dedicated team ready to overcome challenges and strive for excellence.

7. **Maintain a Positive Attitude**: A positive and hopeful attitude is crucial for successful leadership, especially when facing challenges. Positivity can inspire team members and increase their motivation. Optimistic leaders create a supportive environment that motivates their teams to overcome obstacles.

Renowned leadership expert Zig Ziglar once said, "Your attitude, not your aptitude, will determine your altitude," emphasizing the significance of a positive mindset in achieving success and resilience [13]. By demonstrating optimism, leaders can encourage their teams to stay committed and motivated, even in difficult situations.

Encouraging a positive attitude within the team can foster resilience and adaptability. When leaders approach challenges with optimism, it motivates team members to view problems as opportunities for growth and learning rather than roadblocks. This shift in mindset can lead to innovative solutions and a proactive problem-solving mindset. As the famous author Norman Vincent Peale famously stated, "Change your thoughts, and you change your world" [14]. By maintaining a positive outlook, leaders can influence the team's mindset, helping them remain resilient and engaged. This enhances team performance and cultivates a healthier, more collaborative, and productive work environment.

8. **Show Empathy**: Understanding and acknowledging the emotions and perspectives of team members are essential for effective leadership. Showing empathy helps create a compassionate and supportive work environment, which is crucial for encouraging team solidarity and collaboration. When leaders authentically demonstrate care for their team's well-being and address their concerns, it builds trust and reinforces relationships. As Brené Brown, a renowned research professor, highlights, "Empathy involves listening, establishing a safe space, withholding judgment, connecting emotionally, and communicating the powerful message that 'You are not alone'" [15]. By embracing empathy, leaders can make their team members feel valued and understood, ultimately enhancing their commitment and motivation.

   Empathy is essential in resolving conflicts and addressing challenges within the team. When leaders show empathy, they can better understand the root causes of conflicts, enabling them to find considerate solutions. Renowned leadership expert Simon Sinek emphasizes that leadership is about caring for those under your guidance [16]. Prioritizing empathy fosters a harmonious work environment where team members feel supported and empowered. This compassionate approach enhances individual well-being and cultivates a culture of mutual respect and collaboration, resulting in tremendous team success.

9. **Promote Work–Life Balance**: Encouraging a healthy work–life balance for the team is essential in establishing a productive and sustainable work atmosphere. Valuing personal time and well-being is crucial in preventing burnout and maintaining high levels of motivation and dedication among employees. Leaders who prioritize work–life balance demonstrate genuine concern for their team's welfare, emphasizing the significance of assisting team members in managing their personal and professional responsibilities and recognizing the necessity of breaks for long-term success.

   When possible, flexible work arrangements can significantly contribute to promoting work–life balance. Flexible schedules, remote work options, and taking time off when needed are practical measures to help team members man-

age their responsibilities more effectively. Richard Branson, a famous businessman and writer, once said, "Take care of your employees, and they'll take care of your business. It's as simple as that" [17]. By offering flexibility and understanding the diverse needs of team members, leaders can create a more accommodating and supportive work environment. This enhances job satisfaction and loyalty and leads to higher productivity and innovation, as team members can better focus and perform at their best when their well-being is prioritized.
10. **Provide Clear Vision and Goals**: Communicating the team and organization's vision and goals is essential for strong leadership. When leaders clearly articulate an inspiring vision, it gives team members a sense of purpose and direction. This shared understanding of the main objectives helps align individual efforts toward common goals, fostering a cohesive and focused team environment. By clearly defining the vision and goals, leaders ensure that everyone is working toward the same goals, enhancing collaboration and reducing the chances of misunderstandings or conflicting objectives. Ensuring that each team member comprehends their role in achieving these goals is vital. When team members understand how their contributions contribute to the bigger picture, they are more likely to feel appreciated and motivated. This clarity also aids in setting expectations, tracking progress, identifying areas for improvement, and celebrating achievements. As leadership expert Stephen Covey wisely pointed out, "The main thing is to keep the main thing the main thing" [8]. By consistently communicating the vision and goals, leaders help their team stay focused on what truly matters, boosting productivity and achieving better results. Providing clear guidance unites the team and empowers each member to take responsibility for their tasks, knowing that their efforts are essential to the organization's overall success.

Showcasing unwavering commitment to these essential components daily is key to physician leaders creating a culture of engagement that is indispensable for nurturing a thriving environment. This captivating ambiance is crucial for the growth of physician leaders and the progress of the entire team. Embracing these elements ensures long-lasting success and lifelong solid relationships.

Leading a Multi-Generational Workforce

It can be easy to write-off click-bait articles about Baby Boomers and Gen Zs clashing in the workplace, or clueless Gen-X managers using cringe-inducing slang when trying to motivate younger workers, and Millennials with no motivation who've ruined corporate culture. While the rhetoric in these stories is often heightened to the level of comedy, there are myriad reasons why learning to lead a multigenerational team is crucial skill for leaders in academic medicine. At any given time, there are typically five generations in the American workforce, from young interns or fresh hirers right out of college to retired former leaders who stay on in advisory or emeritus roles. Given the ever-changing nature of this field, we will not go into details here about the personalities, preferences, or blind spots of individual generations. However, there are several unchanging benefits of understanding generational traits employees bring with them.

- *Maximizes Engagement*: Leaders who tailor their approach can address specific needs and motivations that vary among the generations.
- *Improves Retention*: Leaders who accommodate values and goals of each generation are more likely to make them feel valued and engaged, increasing retention.
- *Enhances Communication*: Different generations prefer different forms, lengths, tones, and styles of communications. While all employees must learn to communicate within the parameters of what is conventional for their workplace, by having a leader who can tailor their message to each generation, it can improve clarity and minimize misunderstandings.
- *Encourages Innovation*: Leveraging the differences between generations and encouraging collaboration among colleagues from different groups, encourages creative thinking and can drive innovation.
- *Promotes Flexibility*: A leader who can understand the generational trends can help keep their workforce and teams cutting-edge and competitive. New for the sake of newness and continuing to do something because that's the way it has always been done to limit the creativity and talent of employees.
- Lastly, it is critical that all physicians can understand, empathize, and communicate with patients from any generation, as they will rarely only see patients from one age group.

Understanding and Combating Burnout as a Physician Leader

Physicians are facing increasing levels of burnout, along with concerns like suicide, alcohol use, and divorce, which reflect the intense pressures and demands of their profession. Almost 50% of doctors share that they feel burned out, experiencing emotional exhaustion, depersonalization, and a diminished sense of personal accomplishment [18–20]. This issue is especially common in fields that involve constant, high-stakes decision-making, like surgery, emergency medicine, and critical care. The long hours, emotional challenges of caring for patients, and the administrative responsibilities within the healthcare system all play a major role in this widespread burnout, potentially leading to serious personal and professional impacts.

The mental health struggles that physicians encounter is made even more serious by alarmingly high suicide rates. Studies show that doctors face a higher risk of suicide than the general population, with female physicians particularly vulnerable. For example, female doctors are up to 130% more likely to die by suicide compared to women in other fields, while male physicians have a 40% higher risk than their male counterparts in different professions [21]. Unfortunately, the stigma surrounding mental health within the medical field often stops physicians from getting the support they need, resulting in untreated mental health struggles and a heightened risk of suicide. In addition to mental health challenges, doctors frequently encounter other issues such as alcohol use disorder and divorce. Research indicates that physicians are more prone to alcohol use disorder compared to the general population, with approximately 15% admitting to problematic drinking [22]. The high stress and demands of their jobs can also lead to increased divorce rates, as long hours and emotional pressures take a toll on personal relationships [23]. Tackling these challenges calls for a comprehensive approach that includes systemic changes in healthcare and a cultural shift to lessen the stigma around seeking mental health support, while also promoting wellness and resilience among physician leaders.

Physician leaders encounter different stressors in their everyday lives that can lead to a lack of engagement and ultimately burnout. Recognizing these stressors is crucial for physician leaders to address and prevent burnout for themselves and their teams. These stressors fall into four categories: personal, patient-related, organizational, and other professional (Fig. 7.1).

Striking a balance between physician workload and feeling supported is essential for cultivating physician wellness. This support can be broken down into the following areas:

1. **Organizational Support**: Organizational support is crucial for the well-being and effectiveness of physicians in medical practice. Supplying essential resources

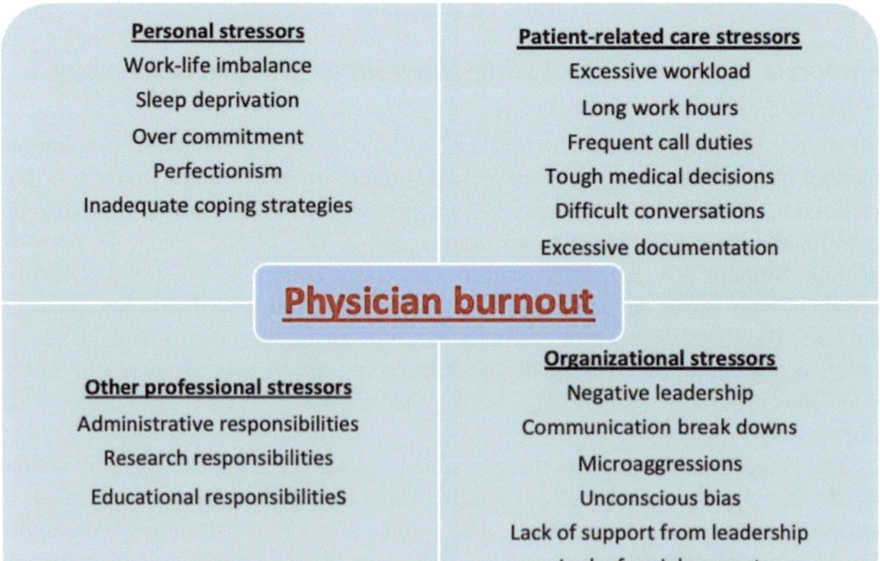

Fig. 7.1 Stressors leading to physician burnout in academic medical centers

such as medical equipment, pagers, computers, and phones ensures that physicians can provide excellent care. These tools streamline patient management, allowing physicians to focus on clinical decision-making rather than administrative tasks. Proper training in electronic medical records (EMRs) is also vital. EMRs are integral to modern healthcare, and thorough training helps physicians use these systems efficiently, reducing errors and improving patient outcomes. Timely technical support is essential, too, as quick resolutions to technology issues prevent disruptions in patient care and minimize physician stress. Ensuring physicians have sufficient time to fulfill their duties is crucial to organizational support. Overloaded schedules and unrealistic patient loads can lead to burnout and decreased job satisfaction. Organizations can help physicians maintain a healthy work–life balance by managing workloads effectively and enhancing their well-being and productivity. Moreover, offering fair and competitive compensation is crucial in recognizing and valuing physicians' hard work and dedication. This not only boosts morale but also shows the organization's commitment to meeting its staff's professional and personal needs. With these elements of organizational support in place, physicians are better equipped to excel in their roles, providing high-quality care to patients and positively impacting the healthcare sector.

2. **A Culture of Wellness**: Establishing a culture of well-being within an organization is crucial for its doctors' long-term health and effectiveness. This culture is built on organizational values, attitudes, and behaviors prioritizing self-care, personal growth, and professional development. Leadership plays a crucial role in setting the tone by recognizing and promoting the importance of well-being. This includes implementing policies that encourage breaks, reasonable work hours, and access to mental health resources. Promoting physical health through fitness initiatives, healthy food options, and ergonomic work environments can significantly enhance overall well-being. By embedding these values at the core of the company, leaders can create an environment where self-care is not just accepted but actively encouraged. A wellness culture extends beyond physical health to encompass emotional and professional development. Organizations should offer opportunities for learning and career progression to support their doctors. This may include access to conferences, workshops, and specialized training programs. Building a supportive community where doctors can share experiences and challenges openly and without judgment is equally essential. Encouraging transparent communication and peer support networks helps cultivate resilience and a sense of belonging. By nurturing a wellness culture, organizations ensure doctors are well equipped for their roles and feel inspired and satisfied.
3. **Developing Resilience**: Resilience involves effectively managing challenging situations positively and flexibly. It is crucial to prioritize the development of resilience in physicians, who face daily stressors as frontline workers. Building resilience enables healthcare professionals to recover quickly from stress and become stronger. This adaptability is essential for their well-being and for providing excellent patient care. Nurturing resilience in physicians involves culti-

vating various essential qualities and abilities to help them cope with job pressures effectively. Resilience is built on three key elements: self-awareness, self-limitation, and public awareness. Recognizing one's weaknesses and emotions is vital for managing stress. Physicians must understand their emotional reactions and know when to step back to prevent burnout. Self-limitation includes recognizing personal boundaries and seeking assistance when necessary. While physicians are accustomed to handling challenging tasks, it is essential to acknowledge limits and ask for help when needed. Public awareness acknowledges the critical role physicians hold in medical organizations. Enhancing understanding of their responsibilities is crucial for fostering solid patient–physician relationships and supporting physician well-being. By focusing on these aspects, organizations can assist physicians in navigating the challenges of their work environment.

The well-being and professional fulfillment of physicians is a vital and intricate matter, influenced by their resilience and the support and environment provided by healthcare institutions (Fig. 7.2). Physicians are highly skilled and adaptable professionals, yet they face significant challenges due to the demanding nature of their roles. As highlighted in the Stanford Model of Professional Fulfillment (Fig. 7.2), healthcare institutions need to go beyond acknowledging these challenges and actively create environments that foster these indispensable team members' mental, emotional, and physical well-being.

Healthcare institutions must invest in robust support systems to bolster physician well-being. This includes offering robust mental health resources to help physicians navigate stress and prevent burnout. Facilitating avenues for professional development is equally crucial, enabling physicians to advance in their careers and elevate job satisfaction. Moreover, cultivating a workplace culture that champions balance and self-care is paramount. This involves implementing initiatives such as flexible scheduling and wellness programs. The commitment to physician wellness should be deeply embedded in the organization's ethos and operations, ensuring that physicians feel appreciated, supported, and equipped to deliver effective patient care. By prioritizing these elements, healthcare organizations can cultivate a sustainable and positive work environment for physicians, ultimately leading to enhanced patient care and organizational prosperity.

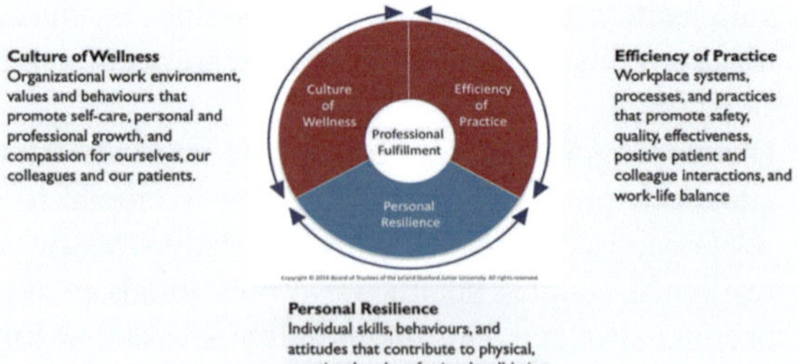

Fig. 7.2 The Stanford model of professional fulfillment

Conclusions

In conclusion, taking care of physicians' well-being is multifaceted and requires a comprehensive strategy. By promoting a culture of engagement and tackling burnout preemptively, healthcare institutions can establish a supportive and enduring workplace. This enhances physicians' well-being, improves patient results, and boosts organizational success. As physician leaders, it's crucial to cultivate an engaging atmosphere while being mindful of personal burnout and that of the team.

Take-Home Points

- Develop and understand a culture of engagement.
- Identify critical components of an engaging culture.
- Recognize factors affecting physician leaders' wellness.
- Address burnout at both personal and organizational levels.

References

1. Maxwell JC. The 21 irrefutable laws of leadership: follow them and people will follow you. Thomas Nelson; 1998.
2. Maxwell JC. Becoming a person of influence: how to positively impact the lives of others. HarperCollins Leadership; 2006.
3. Drucker PF. Management challenges for the 21st century. 1st ed; 2001. HarperBusiness
4. Aziz F, Djamali KS. Providing feedback is essential for professional growth. WMJ. 2023;122(4):238–9. https://www.ncbi.nlm.nih.gov/pubmed/37768759.
5. Wooden J. Wooden on leadership: how to create a winning organization. McGraw Hill; 2005.
6. Carnegie D. How to win friends & influence people. Pocket Books; 1998.
7. Angelou M. Celebrations: rituals of peace and prayer. Random House; 2006.
8. Covey SR. The 7 habits of highly effective people: powerful lessons in personal change. Free Press; 2004.
9. Maxwell JC. The Maxwell Daily Reader: 365 days of insight to develop the leader within you and influence those around you. Thomas Nelson; 2011.
10. Gandhi MK. Gandhi: an autobiography—the story of my experiments with truth. Beacon Press; 1993.
11. Maxwell JC. The 21 indispensable qualities of a leader: becoming the person others will want to follow. Thomas Nelson; 1999.
12. Roosevelt T. Theodore Roosevelt: an autobiography. Macmillan; 1913.
13. Ziglar Z. See you at the top. Pelican; 2006.
14. Peale NV. The power of positive thinking. Prentice-Hall Inc.; 1956.
15. Brown B. Daring greatly: how the courage to be vulnerable transforms the way we live, love, parent, and lead. Avery; 2015.
16. Sinek S. Start with why: how great leaders inspire everyone to take action. Portfolio; 2011.
17. Branson R. The virgin way: everything I know about leadership. Portfolio; 2014.
18. Shanafelt TD, Boone S, Tan L, Dyrbye LN, Sotile W, Satele D, West CP, Sloan J, Oreskovich MR. Burnout and satisfaction with work-life balance among US physicians relative to the

general US population. Arch Intern Med. 2012;172(18):1377–85. https://doi.org/10.1001/archinternmed.2012.3199.
19. Shanafelt TD, Hasan O, Dyrbye LN, Sinsky C, Satele D, Sloan J, West CP. Changes in burnout and satisfaction with work-life balance in physicians and the general US working population between 2011 and 2014. Mayo Clin Proc. 2015;90(12):1600–13. https://doi.org/10.1016/j.mayocp.2015.08.023.
20. Shanafelt TD, Noseworthy JH. Executive leadership and physician well-being: nine organizational strategies to promote engagement and reduce burnout. Mayo Clin Proc. 2017;92(1):129–46. https://doi.org/10.1016/j.mayocp.2016.10.004.
21. Schernhammer ES, Colditz GA. Suicide rates among physicians: a quantitative and gender assessment (meta-analysis). Am J Psychiatry. 2004;161(12):2295–302. https://doi.org/10.1176/appi.ajp.161.12.2295.
22. Gold KJ, Sen A, Schwenk TL. Details on suicide among US physicians: data from the National Violent Death Reporting System. Gen Hosp Psychiatry. 2013;35(1):45–9. https://doi.org/10.1016/j.genhosppsych.2012.08.005.
23. Gabbard GO, Menninger RW. The psychology of postponement in the medical marriage. JAMA. 1989;261(16):2378–81. https://www.ncbi.nlm.nih.gov/pubmed/2704090.

Chapter 8
Feedback in Academic Medicine

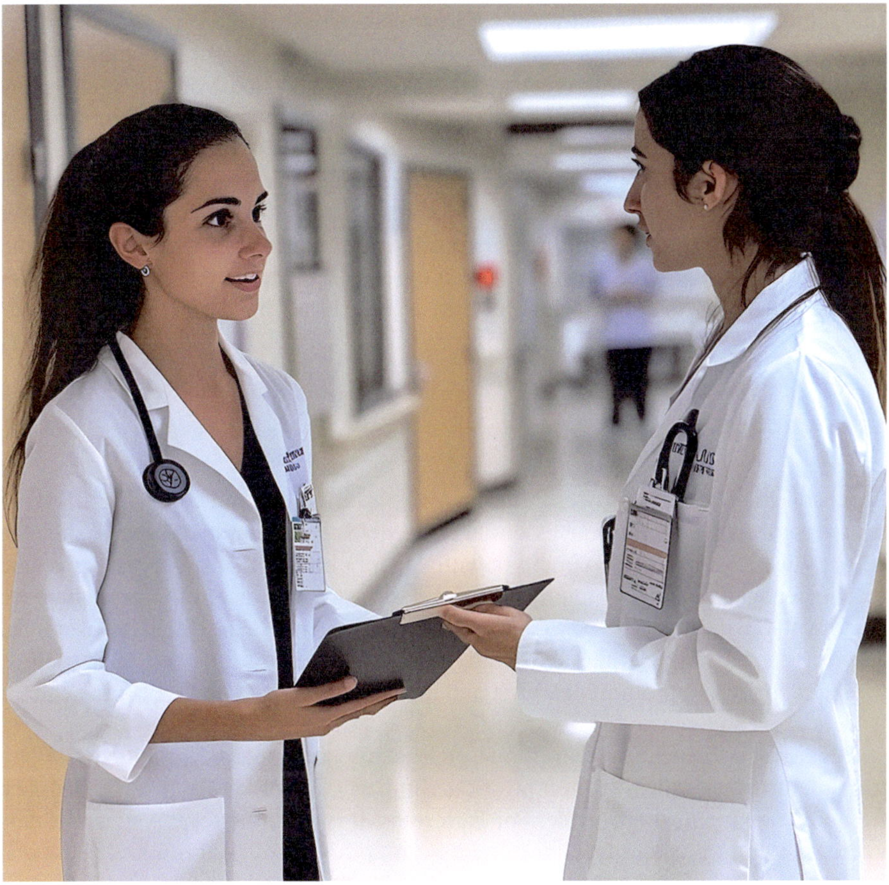

A. Djamali et al., *Emerging Leaders in Academic Medicine*,
https://doi.org/10.1007/978-3-031-80358-1_8

Case Presentation

Dr. Rodriguez is an accomplished endocrinologist who recently transitioned into a leadership role in her division. While her clinical expertise is unquestionable, she faces unique challenges in her new position. Dr. Rodriguez reached out to a trusted mentor expressing her fears and excitement in taking on this leadership work, and her mentor suggested she request a 360 evaluation and coaching session to get a full picture of her situation, strengths, and weaknesses.

Dr. Rodriguez's 360° feedback assessment involved input from colleagues, bosses, supervisees, nurses, and administrative staff. She then met with a leadership coach from her institution who walked her through the feedback, both positive (clinical acumen, delegation) and areas of improvement (strategic planning, transparency). The coach was able to work with Dr. Rodriguez to incorporate this feedback into defining her leadership vision based on her strengths and working in areas that were identified for growth and do so in a way that helped Dr. Rodgriguez build relationships with her team and create transparency and buy-in.

As a result of this 360 assessment and follow-up coaching, Dr. Rodriguez was able to develop her leadership style and skills. This allowed her to empower her team, delegate effectively, and foster a positive and transparent work environment. She also understands the power of receiving and implementing feedback for her own personal growth and development, as well as that of her team.

Introduction

Feedback is a dynamic process that involves both giving and receiving. Hesketh et al. described feedback as an essential element of the educational process that can help trainees reach their maximum potential [1]. Learning how to properly give and receive feedback is critical to physician leaders, as it helps us grow from where we are to where we want to be (see Chap. 1). In academic medicine, feedback is crucial at every career stage, as the stakes are high and the margin for mistakes is low; feedback is vital to promote learning and meet evolving standards. Feedback helps leaders grow and evolve [2].

Feedback is beneficial to everyone on a team and should be provided to every team member, regardless of their position. Similarly, it is crucial to receive feedback from all team members regardless of their roles. It is essential for physician leaders to create a culture where feedback is the norm, praise is offered routinely, and difficult conversations can occur around factual feedback and not personal criticism. This chapter is focused on helping physician leaders develop an approach to giving and receiving feedback. It is divided into two parts: the first will focus on providing effective feedback, and the second will focus on receiving constructive feedback.

Giving Feedback

Physician leaders must understand the difference between feedback that is indirect and too soft to effectively communicate the point and feedback that is too direct and so harsh that it overshadows the point, likely to evoke a negative response from the person receiving it. For effective and constructive feedback, leaders must balance between the two extremes and tailor the style of deliver to the individual based on their personality and listening styles. The more we understand about own personalities, communication preferences, conflict styles, and ourselves as leaders (as discussed in Chaps. 1–3) the better able we will be to provide actionable and effective feedback [3].

Importance of Providing Effective Feedback

Feedback is essential for the growth of young physicians. It is a powerful tool to provide them with nonemotional, fact-based assessment of their performance, assisting them in improving on their weaknesses and encouraging them to grow their strengths. Feedback is vital for the following reasons:

1. Knowledge development
2. Skill development
3. Leadership development
4. Behavioral adjustment to promote team cohesion

Feedback is an integral part of learning. It informs the person of their overall progress and how they can improve. Properly delivered feedback encourages people to take appropriate steps for continued success.

Principles of Providing Feedback

Providing any kind of feedback should be based on the following essential principles. Following these principles makes giving negative feedback easier and helps create a neutral environment for the feedback to be heard.

1. **Keep Calm**: Physician leaders should keep calm during conversations regardless of how crucial or negative the feedback is. It is important to understand that feedback is critical for people to grow, and losing their temperament will not help with the primary goal [4].
2. **Be Specific**: Physician leaders should be specific with any feedback, regardless of how positive or negative it is. Specific data points should be used, and blur words ("always," "often," "never, etc.") should be avoided. It is easy for a recipient to become unsure of what behavior or action to continue or stop when generalized statements are used.

3. **Show the Impact**: Leaders should be able to connect how a specific problem affects the people around them and their own growth. Sometimes making people imagine the impact of the problem helps them to correct it. Likewise, a leader may be able to show a team member the impact of their great work at a higher level than they may have been able to see themselves.
4. **Provide Actionable Solutions**: Feedback without providing actionable items will ultimately be fruitless. Further, giving actionable items provides a measurable response, which is often a requirement if the feedback revolves around a behavioral issue.
5. **Allow Explaining and Active Listening**: By the end of the conversation, people should be allowed to offer their perspective on the issue, as well as share their thoughts on what they think about the feedback. During this time, it is crucial for a leader to stay actively engaged in the conversation and take in what the recipient is saying.

Essential Steps in Providing Feedback

While providing feedback is crucial in academic medicine, physician leaders are rarely given formal training in providing constructive and effective feedback. We suggest the following steps to provide effective feedback based on the above-mentioned principles.

1. **Structure the Feedback**: Feedback must be thoroughly thought through before being shared. We must remember that the purpose of feedback is to help others grow and succeed and to find solutions to any problems. Feedback is not about winning or losing arguments but rather about creating a win–win situation for the person, the team, and the leaders. Before giving feedback, think about the following:

   - **Timing**: When is the right time to provide the input? To the extent possible, the right time for feedback is when everyone's emotions are calm and no one is still in the heat of the moment.
   - **Location**: Where is the right place to share the feedback? Feedback should be provided on a one-on-one basis. Avoid giving feedback in front of other people when possible. People are more receptive to input when provided one-on-one.
   - **Environment**: Make sure there are no distractions while providing feedback. Avoid multitasking while discussing feedback.
   - **Wording**: Carefully formulate the wording. Avoid using aggressive or vague language. Every word should be chosen carefully.
   - **Tone/Body Language**: Use a nonjudgmental, fact-based approach to giving feedback. Body language should be relaxed and nonaggressive.

2. **Tailor the Feedback to the Specific Recipient**: Feedback should be tailored to the individual, considering their personality and preferred method of communication.

3. **Be Specific in Constructive Feedback**: To avoid confusion, physician leaders should be specific and nonjudgmental in their negative feedback. Providing objective data rather than subjective information, focusing on specific incidents rather than generalized statements. Understanding how this can affect the people around them and their growth is essential, as it will provide them with a reason to obtain further constructive feedback.
4. **Provide Feedback on Improving Shortcomings**: Feedback without clear, actionable items can be confusing and often fruitless. Physician leaders should provide actionable items on improving the specific problem. It's also essential to provide a roadmap of the solutions and allow leaders to track progress.
5. **Make Yourself Available to Answer Questions**: Leaders should always make themselves available to answer any questions regarding the feedback and the actionable items. Answering questions helps to clear up any confusion and helps them understand that the leader is genuinely invested in their progress and growth.

Things to Avoid in Providing Feedback

Physician leaders should avoid a few things while providing feedback. These are given in Table 8.1.

Barriers to Providing Constructive Feedback

Physician leaders need to understand the barriers to providing constructive and effective feedback. Overcoming these barriers helps us to develop a strategy to give meaningful feedback.

1. **Fear of Offending the Other Person**: Sometimes the fear of offending the other person causes a person to deliver a muddled message (sugar-coating negative feedback with positive, for example), rendering the feedback ineffective. This fear can be mitigated by learning and using the principles and steps outlined above.
2. **Afraid of Outcomes**: Sometimes, the fear of the outcome prevents physician leaders from giving effective feedback. This barrier can easily be overcome if we

Table 8.1 Things to avoid while providing feedback

1. Disrespectful attitude and environment
2. Judgmental approach
3. Too general
4. Too detailed
5. Focused on personalities and not issues
6. Not goal-oriented
7. No suggestions for improvement
8. No actionable items
9. No plan for follow-up

remember that feedback is essential for the growth of the whole team as well as the individual person.

3. **Lack of Insight**: A lack of proper understanding can lead to inadequate and inappropriate feedback. Physician leaders should carefully think through the issue before providing feedback.
4. **Assume That People Already Know Your Feedback or Can Read Your Mind**: In our busy days as physician leaders, it is easy to fall into the trap that our team members already know what we think about their work or performance and that feedback conversations are not necessary. This is not true. Whether separate conversations or a standing item incorporated into a recurring 1:1 meeting, regular feedback is critical for the development of both the leader and team member.

   Due to these barriers, and others reviewed in Chap. 1, Fig. 1.2, we may deliver inadequate feedback. After all, we are human beings, even as leaders! For example, during morning rounds, Dr. Adam, who is a senior resident says to Dr. Bean, junior resident: "Your patient presentations are always confusing! I don't understand anything." Well, while the timing of the feedback might have been appropriate, the delivery lacks specificity and actionable items. Now, Dr. Bean is confused and afraid of asking follow-up questions. Dr. Adam notes this confusion and apologizes for the inadequate feedback, clarifying expectations: "I am sorry for not giving you proper feedback. I meant you should start with the chief complaint and then follow up with the history of present illness, past medical history, list of medications and allergies, physical exam and laboratories findings, and finish with your assessment and plan. This morning, for this patient, your presentation started with past medical history and then the history of present illness. Then you talked about the lab results and forgot to mention anything about your clinical exam findings. I am happy to set up a time for the two of us to review your presentation technique after rounds today." Now this feedback is more constructive. In addition, Dr. Adam has apologized, showing vulnerability. This is helpful in building trust in a professional relationship.

Receiving Feedback

Our ability to receive feedback—both complimentary and critical—is foundational for continued success and growth as physician leaders. Embracing feedback, regardless of its nature, reflects a leader's humility and openness to differing perspectives. This receptiveness to feedback is not merely a professional skill but a vital life lesson that underscores the importance of understanding the impact of one's actions and behaviors on others. Showing that we as leaders are receptive to feedback helps create emotional reciprocity with our team members and can help them become better at receiving feedback from us.

Demonstrating how to properly accept feedback is fundamental to our role in creating a culture that values continuous growth and transparent dialogue. Active listening, openness to constructive critique, and a commitment to reflective practice

Table 8.2 Advantages of welcoming feedback

1. Helps leaders grow
2. Increases self-awareness
3. Increases influence with others
4. Improves teamwork
5. Develops a trustworthy environment

enable physician leaders to illustrate to our colleagues the significance of feedback as an instrument for both personal and collective development. Such a strategy not only cultivates a conducive atmosphere for learning but also bolsters mutual respect and teamwork. When physician leaders welcome feedback with modesty and willingness to evolve, they catalyze improvements in patient care, team cohesion, and the overall resilience of the healthcare system. By setting a robust example in the art of feedback reception, we can highlight that feedback transcends routine procedure—it is an indispensable element of clinical prowess and leadership.

Taking feedback effectively has several advantages. A few are given in Table 8.2.

Principles of Receiving Feedback

Receiving feedback should be based on the following five essential principles:

(a) **Actively Ask for Feedback**: Physician leaders should actively ask for feedback. It should be requested not only from senior leaders but also from peers and those who are more junior. Asking for feedback shows how seriously you are interested in improving yourself and helps establish that feedback is an expected part of being a team member.

(b) **Radical Listening to Feedback**: While receiving feedback, radical listening is essential. This includes understanding every word, the meaning of every word, the meaning between the lines, and body language. Radical listening is a necessary component of self-improvement.

(c) **Ask a Question**: Always ask questions to better understand the feedback. Good questions can provide clarity and demonstrate your commitment to the feedback process.

(d) **Ask for Actionable Items**: Always ask for actionable items based on the feedback. Feedback without actionable items rarely results in change.

(e) **Act on the Feedback**: Acting positively on constructive feedback with a growth mindset is essential. A growth mindset approach to feedback helps leaders grow.

Essential Steps in Taking Feedback

Taking in feedback with a growth mindset is essential for the growth of physician leaders; however, formal training is rarely given on receiving feedback and using it constructively. We suggest the following steps to receive feedback effectively based on the above-mentioned principles.

1. **Connect with the People Around You and Ask for Feedback**: Actively letting those you work with know you are very open to feedback is critical to our development as physician leaders. Asking for both positive and negative feedback is essential, and we should solicit this input from all those around us, including those working for us, our peers, and our superiors.
2. **Take Positive Feedback Wisely**: Positive feedback guides us on what we are doing well and what we should do more of. Recognizing our strengths through positive feedback is essential; however, we should not become complacent in our development because we are already doing some things well.
3. **Take Negative Feedback Constructively**: Negative feedback can be stressful. However, even negative feedback should be taken with a growth mindset, as it guides us on how to improve ourselves.
4. **Keep Emotions Calm**: Regardless of the feedback and whether we like it, it is essential to keep ourselves from acting on these emotions. It is also important to ask for clarification so that we can develop a better understanding of the negative feedback. Just as we remind our employees that feedback is about finding a win–win, so too must we remember this if we receive negative feedback that might not feel good [4].
5. **Always Ask for Actionable Items and Roadmap**: After receiving feedback, if it's not already given, we should ask for actionable items for how to use the feedback constructively. After getting the feedback and the actionable items, we should develop a roadmap to improve the weaknesses and strengthen the positives.
6. **Work on the Feedback**: After getting any feedback, we must act on it and improve ourselves. Taking feedback and not working on it sends the message that we are not interested in what our employees, peers, or superiors think and are not interested in our own development.

Things to Avoid in Receiving Feedback

Physician leaders should avoid a few things while receiving feedback. These are given in Table 8.3.

Table 8.3 Things to avoid while receiving feedback

1. Passively waiting for feedback
2. Only taking input from specific people
3. Acting defensively
4. Not analyzing feedback
5. Not asking for actionable items
6. Not acting on feedback

Conclusion

Providing and receiving feedback is crucial for the growth of the physician leaders and the success of our teams. Incorporating feedback effectively is a dynamic process where leaders take the initiative to provide and receive feedback and encourage team members to do the same. We must be mindful that feedback without providing actionable items for change or growth is often fruitless.

Take-Home Points

- Cultivating an atmosphere of providing feedback is imperative for physician leaders to construct robust teams with an attitude of personal development and team unity.
- Actively seeking out feedback allows us to develop ourselves as physician leaders.
- Physician leaders recognize the significance of cultivating an environment in which providing and receiving feedback is an integral part of the culture.

References

1. Hesketh EA, Laidlaw JM. Developing the teaching instinct, 1: feedback. Med Teach. 2002;24(3):245–8. https://doi.org/10.1080/01421590220140991 1.
2. Aziz F, Djamali KS. Providing feedback is essential for professional growth. WMJ. 2023;122(4):238–9. https://www.ncbi.nlm.nih.gov/pubmed/37768759.
3. Overton AR, Lowry AC. Conflict management: difficult conversations with difficult people. Clin Colon Rectal Surg. 2013;26(4):259–64. https://doi.org/10.1055/s-0033-1356728.
4. Abrams H. Holding the calm: the secret to resolving conflict and defusing tension. Berrett-Koehler Publishers; 2020.

Chapter 9
Mentorship

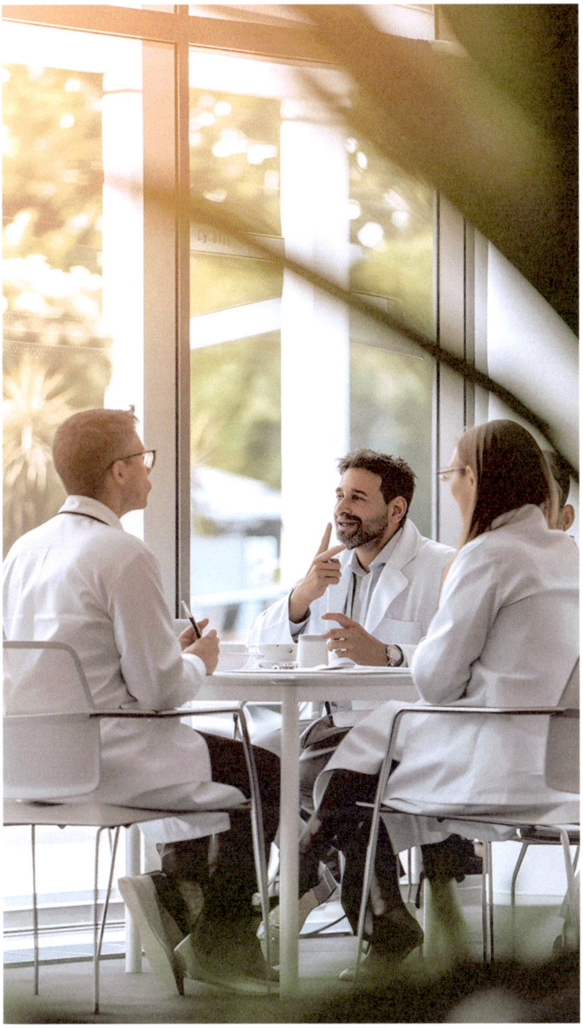

A. Djamali et al., *Emerging Leaders in Academic Medicine*,
https://doi.org/10.1007/978-3-031-80358-1_9

Case Presentation

Dr. Khan is a male physician and assistant professor at an academic medical center who is currently on the unmodified/tenure track. Because of his track record and area of specialization, he was hired with protected time for research, grant applications, and publications. He was also automatically enrolled in his department's mentoring program and assigned a mentor.

Dr. Khan spends the first year of his career building his lab, beginning experiments, and generally settling into life on the tenure track. He meets regularly with his mentor, and they create a plan for academic output and progressive goals toward promotion. Despite this plan and regular mentoring meetings, Dr. Khan submits limited publications and few grant applications during the next 2 years. Excuses abound and mentoring meetings become increasingly unproductive, ultimately resulting in Dr. Khan terminating the mentoring relationship. Dr. Khan's fourth and fifth years are spent scrambling as he continues to struggle to turn his research into any scholarly product. After another year spent without major publications or securing extramural funding, Dr. Khan's promotion on the unmodified/tenure track is rejected, and he is forced to leave the institution and change to a clinical career in private practice.

While Dr. Khan's promotion denial is multifactorial and the result of leaving academic medicine is extreme, it provides an illustrative example of what can happen when mentoring relationships break down and how difficult it is to navigate a career in academic medicine on one's own.

Introduction

Mentoring is a relationship where a more experienced or knowledgeable person guides, advises, and supports a less experienced individual to help develop the junior person in a specific area. Professional benefits of mentoring include, though certainly are not limited to, knowledge transfer, career advancement, skill development, networking, emotional support, and providing a springboard to independence. When mentoring is successful, it also fosters personal growth, accelerates learning, and provides insights and perspective from someone with shared experience.

Mentorship is an invaluable part of our growth and development as physician leaders. When beginning a position at a new institution, one of the biggest ways we can position ourselves for success is to seek out a mentor. It is important to remember that mentors don't hold all the answers to all areas of our careers, and it is often appropriate to have multiple mentors at one time. This is not so we can opinion shop and play them against each other to hear only what we want but rather so that they can provide expert knowledge and experience in the different areas of our career (research mentor, academic career/trajectory; clinical leadership, etc.). The more we actively engage in being a mentee, the more we can offer junior faculty in the future when we ourselves become mentors.

Why Engage in Mentorship?

There are many reasons to engage in mentorship [1]:

1. **Career Development**: In academic medicine, career paths can be complex and competitive. Mentoring provides guidance on how to navigate these paths and make informed decisions about research, clinical work, and teaching. Mentors guide you in developing competencies essential for professional growth, can open doors to new opportunities, and help overcome career obstacles by sharing their experiences and providing advice. Learning from their wisdom saves you from trial and error. They assist in setting and achieving career goals, offering insights into specific professions or organizations, and helping you strategize and navigate your unique path.
2. **Skill Development and Transfer of Knowledge**: Mentors play a pivotal role in both skill development and knowledge transfer and provide personalized guidance for a trainee to enhance specific skills. They can help mentees develop in all aspects of their careers, whether specific task-related skills when conducting research, publishing papers, or effective teaching methods to more concept-based skills such as communication, problem-solving, or leadership. In terms of knowledge transfer, mentors pass on their wisdom, experiences, and lessons learned. This includes industry-specific knowledge, best practices, and problem-solving techniques. Encouragement and acknowledgment from mentors boost mentees' self-confidence, and constructive feedback from mentors helps mentees refine their abilities. Overall, mentoring fosters a positive organizational culture where knowledge flows freely and creates depth and loyalty within the organization. Remember, a mentor isn't just a teacher—they're a catalyst for growth and success.
3. **Networking**: Mentors play a pivotal role in expanding your professional network, both by introducing you to key people in their network and by sharing their own effective networking techniques—how to reach out, build relationships, and maintain connections. Leveraging your mentor's network is an economical way to connect with influential individuals who can offer insights and opportunities. Through your mentor, you'll be introduced to the right circles—people who can enhance your career and broaden your horizons. These introductions often happen at networking events, seminars, or professional associations. Mentors also provide encouragement, nudging you to attend events, join industry groups, and connect with relevant professionals. Mentorship isn't just about skills; it's about expanding your professional universe.
4. **Feedback and Support**: Mentors play a pivotal role in providing feedback and support to their mentees. Effective mentors start with positive reinforcement. They highlight what you're doing well, reinforcing your strengths and boosting confidence. Instead of vague feedback, mentors use specific examples when it comes to areas of improvement. They encourage you to reflect on your performance and goals. This self-awareness fosters growth. Mentors offer guidance, advice, and resources. They share insights from their experiences, helping you

navigate challenges. Their support extends beyond technical skills—it includes emotional encouragement and motivation. A mentor's feedback and support create a nurturing environment for your professional development.

5. **Professional Identity and Values**: Mentoring can help shape a mentee's professional identity and values. Mentors serve as role models, demonstrating professionalism, ethics, and integrity. By observing their mentor's behavior, mentees learn valuable lessons about how to navigate the professional world. Mentors provide constructive feedback, encouraging mentees to reflect on their actions, decisions, and values. This self-awareness helps shape their professional identity and in turn helps guide their choices, interactions, and ethical behavior in the workplace. Remember, mentorship isn't just about receiving guidance; it's about actively engaging in the process of shaping one's leadership identity. Mentees are encouraged to reflect on their experiences, recognize their strengths, and identify areas for improvement. By doing so, they can effectively leverage the wisdom and insights of their mentors.
6. **Retention and Satisfaction**: Effective mentoring can enhance job satisfaction and reduce burnout among academic medicine professionals. Mentors play a pivotal role in employee retention and job satisfaction. Mentors act as a sounding board, offering both professional guidance and personal support. This reaffirms the employee's value to the organization, enhancing job satisfaction and engagement. Mentoring provides a clear path for development within the company. It opens up opportunities for employees to achieve their career goals while fostering loyalty to the organization. Remember, mentorship goes beyond skill development—it creates a sense of value and appreciation among staff members!
7. **Diversity and Inclusion**: Mentoring plays a critical role in promoting diversity and inclusion in academic medicine. Mentor–mentee pairings that cross cultural, racial, gender, and other demographic lines break down barriers and foster understanding. Mentors offer equitable access to experienced professionals, helping underrepresented groups find guidance, support, and career opportunities. Through personal interactions, mentors foster empathy and expose both parties to new viewpoints. This contributes to an inclusive mindset and behavior. Mentors create an environment where diverse perspectives are acknowledged, valued, and integrated into the organizational fabric. Mentorship isn't just about skills—it's a catalyst for positive change and growth.

Understanding Your Institution's Mentoring Opportunities

Although the principles of mentoring are constant, mentoring programs can vary widely among institutions. Some offer formal programs for all junior faculty, some only for tenure-track faculty, and some only in certain areas (research but not in education). You are your own best advocate when it comes to mentoring—do not be shy about asking your leader or more senior faculty members for advice finding a mentor. Learn what the mentoring culture and opportunities are at your institution, and volunteer for committee service in areas of your interest to make connections with faculty who share similar interests to yours.

Mentoring relationships can be both formal and informal; however, there are some general principles that apply to both types that will help set you up for success. It is critical that expectations align for both the mentor and mentee and that you share an understanding of the details about the mentoring relationship.

The Mentoring Cycle/Phases

The mentoring cycle is the natural progression of the mentoring relationship.

According to the National Institute of Health Science Research, the five stages of the mentoring relationship are[1]:

1. **Rapport Building**: The rapport-building stage in a mentoring relationship is the initial phase where the mentor and mentee establish a positive connection. During this stage, they engage in dialogue to determine if they can work productively together and involves setting goals, clarifying expectations, and building rapport between mentor and mentee. Key factors for building rapport include alignment of values, mutual respect, and clear expectations regarding roles and behaviors. Effective mentors actively listen, show genuine interest, and demonstrate empathy to foster a sense of psychological safety, which is crucial for open communication.
2. **Setting Direction**: After establishing rapport, this stage involves identifying the mentee's goals and what they wish to achieve with the mentor's support. It sets the course for their collaboration, ensuring alignment and purpose. The mentor provides guidance, support, and resources for the mentee to tackle the problem and work toward identified goals.
3. **Progression**: The progression phase in a mentoring relationship is where the mentee begins making significant strides toward their goals. This is where the hard work for the mentee begins and will involve successes, but also often challenges and obstacles, and sometimes even failure. Feedback and self-reflection are integral to the success of this step. It's a critical stage for growth and opportunity.
4. **Winding Down**: The winding down phase of a mentoring relationship occurs as goals are met, signaling the eventual closure of the formal mentor–mentee connection. During this stage, both mentor and mentee prepare for the transition. Mentors focus on ensuring the mentee's future success, which may involve solidifying their network or establishing a path for continued growth. Celebrating achievements and reviewing progress are essential aspects of this phase.
5. **Moving On**: The moving on phase in a mentoring relationship marks its closure. During this stage, the mentee and mentor formally end their structured mentor-

[1] Phases of the mentoring relationship | NIHR

ship and may transition to a more informal friendship or professional relationship. It's essential because it allows both parties to reflect on progress, celebrate achievements, and prepare for independent growth.

Being a Mentee

Being a good mentee is essential for making the most out of a mentoring relationship and maximizing your personal and professional development. Here are some key tips on how to be a good mentee:

1. **Clarify and Specify Your Goals**: Before entering into a mentoring relationship, have a clear understanding of what you hope to achieve. Define your goals, both short term and long term. Once you have a mentor, communicate these goals clearly to your mentor. Setting clear goals as a mentee is crucial for several reasons. Clearly defined goals help you understand what you want to achieve from the mentoring relationship. They guide your efforts and resources toward specific outcomes, making your learning journey more purposeful and effective. Goal-setting encourages you to step out of your comfort zone and embrace new challenges. As you work toward your goals, you acquire new knowledge, skills, and experiences that contribute to your overall professional development. Additionally, when you set clear goals, you establish measurable milestones to track your progress. This accountability helps you manage your time effectively and stay motivated as you work toward your desired outcomes.
2. **Respect Your Mentor's Time**: Be mindful of your mentor's time and commitments. Come prepared for meetings, stick to scheduled times, and be respectful of their availability. Respecting your mentor's time is crucial for a successful mentor–mentee relationship. Recognize that your mentor voluntarily invests their precious time to guide you. Show appreciation by being punctual for meetings and respecting their schedule; avoid last-minute cancellations without valid reasons. Being ready to focus during sessions demonstrates your commitment and respect. A considerate approach fosters a positive and productive mentoring experience.
3. **Be Organized**: Being organized is crucial for mentees for several reasons. A structured approach to personal development involves identifying areas for improvement, setting specific, measurable goals, seeking feedback, reflecting on progress, and celebrating milestones. This organization helps transform mentorship experiences into substantial growth opportunities. This organization can help you stay on track and make the most of your mentor's guidance. It helps them track progress and maintain focus, preventing them from forgetting their objectives. Organized mentees manage their time effectively, making the most of their mentor's guidance. They can prioritize tasks, streamline processes, and optimize their learning journey.

4. **Be Open to Feedback**: Being open to feedback as a mentee is crucial for several reasons. Feedback helps you identify areas for improvement. Honest feedback builds trust while challenging your preconceptions and existing habits, allowing you to grow and change effectively. Quality feedback balances criticism with validation. Celebrating successes while addressing weaknesses ensures a healthy mentoring relationship. Understand that feedback is a valuable tool for growth and improvement.
5. **Actively Seek Guidance**: Don't wait for your mentor to initiate every interaction. Take the initiative to reach out, ask questions, and seek guidance when you encounter challenges or need advice. If helpful, set recurring mentoring meetings at the beginning of the mentoring relationship to build the habit. Your success demonstrates their value to others. Active engagement and reflection enhance your growth as a mentee. Seek mentors aligned with your learning objectives and career aspirations.
6. **Listen and Learn**: Pay close attention to your mentor's advice, experiences, and insights. Actively listen, ask questions for clarification, and show that you value their wisdom. Listening to a mentor's advice is essential for your growth as a mentee. Mentors often have years of experience in their field. Their insights can help you avoid common pitfalls and navigate challenges. Mentors provide an external viewpoint. They can see patterns and opportunities that you might miss due to your proximity to the situation. Mentors share their own failures and lessons learned. You can benefit from their experiences without making the same errors. When you follow their advice, you demonstrate commitment and respect. It also helps build trust between you and your mentor. Active listening and thoughtful consideration of their advice lead to meaningful progress.
7. **Take Responsibility for Your Development**: While your mentor can provide guidance, it's ultimately your responsibility to act on their advice and work toward your goals. Taking responsibility for your own development as a mentee is crucial for several reasons. By actively participating in your growth, you demonstrate commitment and initiative. You become an active learner rather than a passive recipient of advice. You can tailor your learning journey to your specific needs and goals. You know your strengths, weaknesses, and preferences better than anyone else. Reflecting on your progress helps you identify areas for improvement. You can adjust your strategies and seek relevant guidance. When you take charge of your development, you empower yourself. Ownership ensures sustained growth beyond the mentorship period. It's an investment in your future. Active engagement, curiosity, and a growth mindset contribute to your success as a mentee.
8. **Ask for Help When Needed**: Don't hesitate to ask for assistance when you need it. Your mentor is there to support you, and they appreciate when you are proactive in seeking help. Asking for help as a mentee is essential for several reasons. Seeking guidance taps into the collective knowledge and expertise of others. It fosters a sense of interconnectedness and belonging. When you ask for help, you gain insights that can help you solve challenges more effectively and efficiently. It empowers you to access resources beyond your own capabili-

ties, leading to growth and development. Asking for help strengthens relationships and builds trust, creating a culture of reciprocity and collaboration.

9. **Be Patient and Persistent**: Personal and professional growth takes time. Be patient with yourself and persistent in your efforts to achieve your goals. Being persistent as a mentee is crucial for your growth and success, as it helps you push through obstacles. When faced with setbacks, it's essential to stay committed and keep trying. Consistent effort leads to skill improvement. Whether learning a new language or mastering a technical skill, persistence pays off. Mentees who persist develop resilience. They bounce back from failures and setbacks, learning valuable lessons along the way. Long-term goals require sustained effort. Persistence ensures you stay on track and reach your desired outcomes. Your dedication reflects positively on both you and your mentor.
10. **Reflect on Your Progress**: Periodically assess your progress and reflect on what you've learned and accomplished. This self-reflection can help you adjust when needed and set new goals. Reflecting on your progress as a mentee is essential for several reasons. As you evolve, your needs and goals shift. Regular reflection helps you recognize when adjustments are necessary. By assessing your progress, you can make informed decisions. If you're veering off track, reflection allows you to recalibrate. Reflecting on your journey helps consolidate lessons learned. It turns experiences into valuable insights. Self-awareness and introspection contribute to your development and you become more deliberate in your actions. Sharing reflections with your mentor fosters open communication and mutual understanding.
11. **Be Respectful and Show Appreciation**: Expressing genuine gratitude as a mentee is essential for several reasons. Thanking your mentor or mentee fosters a stronger connection. It shows respect and appreciation, enhancing the relationship beyond the mentorship itself. Simple acts like saying "thank you" or offering a token of appreciation contribute to a healthy workplace culture. Feeling appreciated motivates employees and improves overall satisfaction and productivity. Gratitude cements relationships beyond the mentorship period. It establishes mutual respect and can last for years to come.
12. **Communicate Effectively**: Effective communication is key to a successful mentoring relationship. Clear communication fosters trust between mentors and mentees, creating a solid foundation for the relationship. It helps set clear expectations, ensuring both parties are on the same page regarding goals, boundaries, and roles. Through effective communication, mentees can seek guidance, ask questions, and learn from their mentors' experiences. When challenges arise, open communication allows mentees to discuss issues, brainstorm solutions, and adapt strategies. Regular communication enables feedback, reflection, and adjustments, leading to continuous improvement.
13. **Share Your Successes and Challenges**: Keep your mentor informed about your achievements and any obstacles you encounter. Sharing your experiences helps your mentor provide relevant guidance. When mentors convey their successes, mentees can use them as examples to strive toward. They can learn from the steps taken by successful mentors and apply similar strategies to their own

journey. Mentors also share the mistakes they made along their paths. Mentees benefit by learning lessons about the negative impacts of these mistakes without having to suffer the consequences themselves. Openly discussing challenges allows for real-time advice and adjustments. Honest communication ensures alignment with goals and helps navigate obstacles effectively. Remember, transparency and openness contribute to a healthy mentor–mentee relationship.

14. **Show Growth and Improvement**: Demonstrate that you are actively applying the advice and guidance you receive by showing growth and improvement in your skills and knowledge. By believing that abilities can be developed through effort, you view challenges as opportunities for learning. Persisting through setbacks and seeking feedback contribute to your progress. Mentoring helps you develop critical skills like communication, problem-solving, and leadership. Demonstrating growth enhances your chances of achieving your career goals. Sharing your aspirations and setting goals with your mentor allows them to understand your intentions. Your growth benefits not only you but also your organization. Consistent improvement leads to a rewarding mentoring experience and a positive impact for yourself and those you work with by the example you set.

Being a Mentor

Being a good mentor is a rewarding experience that involves providing guidance, support, and encouragement to someone who is seeking to develop personally or professionally. Whether you're mentoring in an academic setting, a workplace, or any other context, here are some key principles and practices to help you become a good mentor:

1. **Establish Clear Expectations**: Clarifying expectations helps both mentors and mentees understand their respective roles, so it is critical to begin the mentoring relationship by discussing goals and expectations with your mentee. What are their objectives? What do they hope to achieve through this mentorship? What can they expect from you as a mentor? What do you expect from them as your mentee? Setting clear expectations is crucial for effective mentorship. When mentors and mentees have well-defined roles and understand their responsibilities, it leads to a more productive and fulfilling relationship. When everyone knows what is expected of them, it reduces confusion and ensures alignment. Clear expectations also create accountability. Mentees know what they need to achieve, and mentors can guide them accordingly. Regular communication and revisiting goals help maintain focus. Having specific goals and expectations streamlines the mentorship process. It helps mentors provide targeted advice and ensures mentees maximize their learning and development. Effective mentorship is a two-way street, and setting expectations lays the foundation for a successful mentoring relationship.

2. **Listen Actively**: Active listening is a vital skill for mentors, fostering effective communication and meaningful relationships. Active listening creates a safe space for mentees to express themselves and allows you to understand their needs, concerns, and aspirations. When you genuinely engage with their thoughts and feelings, trust and respect flourish. Give them your full attention and validate their feelings and experiences. By paying attention to verbal cues, body language, and emotions, mentors can identify underlying issues. This insight leads to better problem-solving and guidance. Active listening helps de-escalate conflicts. When mentors truly understand mentees' perspectives, they can address disagreements constructively. Active listening isn't just about hearing words—it's about connecting on a deeper level and showing empathy.
3. **Build Trust**: When mentors and mentees trust each other, it creates a foundation for open communication, growth, and mutual respect. Novice mentors should speak less and listen more. When mentees feel truly heard, it opens up a magical space in the relationship. Experienced mentors can overcome the urge to dominate conversations and focus on attentive listening. Create an environment where your mentee feels safe sharing their thoughts and concerns. Respect the confidentiality of your mentee's personal and professional matters. They should feel comfortable discussing sensitive topics with you. When mentees trust that their shared information won't become dinner table conversation, they become more vulnerable, which enhances their learning experience. Share your mistakes, weaknesses, and failures. By doing so, you become more approachable and knock yourself off the pedestal, fostering trust. Remember, trust is built over time through consistent actions, empathy, and genuine care for your mentee's growth.
4. **Offer Constructive Feedback**: Providing constructive feedback as a mentor is essential for growth and development and best approached with empathy and genuine concern for a mentee's growth. Clearly state what you noticed and how it affected the mentee or the situation, as feedback should focus on observed actions and their impact. Offer feedback promptly after an event or interaction. Fresh insights are more valuable. Acknowledge your mentor's strengths and contributions, balancing constructive feedback with positive reinforcement. Make it a two-way conversation. Ask questions, seek their perspective, and encourage open dialogue. Ensure they comprehend your feedback and clarify any doubts or misconceptions. Revisit the feedback in subsequent sessions. Monitor progress and adjust as needed.
5. **Share Your Knowledge and Experience**: As a mentor, you enable your mentee's professional and personal development. Draw upon your own experiences and expertise to provide insights, advice, and guidance. Share relevant stories and lessons from your career journey. Sharing your knowledge and experience as a mentor is essential for both your mentee's growth and your own development. By sharing insights, guidance, and expertise, you help them navigate challenges and achieve their goals. Whether it's specific skills, industry know-how, or practical advice, sharing this knowledge accelerates your mentee's

learning curve. This collaboration can help you and your mentee to set clear, achievable goals. Mentorship is a reciprocal relationship where both parties benefit. By sharing your knowledge generously, you contribute to a thriving learning environment.

6. **Set Goals and Action Plans**: Collaborate with your mentee to set achievable goals and create action plans to reach those goals. Monitor progress and adjust as needed. Setting mentoring goals is crucial for both mentors and mentees. It provides direction, enhances the mentoring relationship, and ensures progress. Here's a step-by-step approach:

   - **Define Clear Objectives**: Mentors and mentees should collaboratively set specific, measurable, and achievable goals. These objectives guide the mentoring journey and create a shared vision.
   - **Break Down Goals**: Divide larger goals into smaller, actionable steps. Consider daily, weekly, or monthly milestones. This breakdown helps track progress and maintain focus.
   - **Map Out a Timeline**: Establish deadlines for each milestone. Having a timeline ensures accountability and motivates consistent effort.
   - **Discuss Strategies and Tactics**: Brainstorm strategies to achieve goals. Identify necessary actions, resources, and potential obstacles. Discuss how to overcome challenges.
   - **Monitor Progress**: Regularly assess progress. Adjust strategies if needed. Celebrate achievements and learn from setbacks.

7. **Be Patient and Flexible**: Being patient as a mentor when your mentee faces challenges is essential. Recognize that growth and development take time. Be patient and adaptable to your mentee's pace and changing needs. Understand that everyone learns at their own pace, and struggles are part of the process. Listen attentively to their concerns. Sometimes, sharing their difficulties can alleviate the pressure. Help them break complex tasks into smaller steps. Celebrate progress along the way. Ask questions that prompt them to analyze their struggles. Encourage them to find solutions independently. Remind them that mistakes are opportunities for growth. Share your own experiences of overcoming challenges.
8. **Empower and Encourage Independence**: Encourage your mentee to take ownership of their development and empower them to make decisions and solve problems on their own while you provide guidance when necessary. Guide rather than dictate. Acknowledge their achievements, no matter how small, as positive reinforcement boosts confidence and builds a mentee's autonomy. When they encounter challenges, ask open-ended questions to help them explore solutions independently. Empowering mentees leads to confident, capable individuals.
9. **Provide Resources and Connections**: Offer resources, recommend books or articles, and introduce your mentee to relevant contacts or networks that can help them in their journey.

Resource Sharing:

- **Online Materials**: Share relevant articles, blogs, videos, and tutorials related to their field of interest.
- **Books**: Recommend books or e-books that align with their learning goals.
- **Courses and Workshops**: Point them to online courses, webinars, or workshops.
- **Tools and Software**: Introduce them to tools, software, or apps that enhance their skills.

Networking and Connections:

- **Introduce Them**: Connect them with professionals in their industry. Attend networking events together.
- **LinkedIn**: Encourage them to build a strong LinkedIn profile and connect with relevant contacts.
- **Alumni Networks**: Leverage your own network or their educational institution's alumni network.

10. **Promote Self-Reflection**: Self-awareness is a crucial aspect of personal and professional growth; encourage your mentee to reflect on their experiences, strengths, and areas for improvement. Encouraging self-reflection in your mentee is essential for their growth. Offer constructive feedback that helps them assess their progress and areas for improvement. Encourage mentees to maintain a reflective journal. *Writing* down experiences, challenges, and insights fosters self-awareness and personal discovery. Regularly discuss their progress and challenges. These check-ins create opportunities for reflection and adjustment. When appropriate, pose reflective questions like:

    - "What did you do well?"
    - "What could you improve?"
    - "What will you do differently next time?"

    Self-reflection empowers mentees to learn, adapt, and thrive!
11. **Be a Role Model**: Lead by example in terms of professionalism, ethics, and behavior. Being a positive role model as a mentor is crucial for inspiring and guiding your mentee. Show enthusiasm, resilience, and optimism. Your attitude sets an example for handling challenges and staying productive. Model the behaviors and actions required for success in your field. Be professional, ethical, and respectful. Your mentee will learn from your actions, both job skills and when it comes to traits like self-awareness, empathy, and compassion. These qualities contribute to their overall growth.
12. **Respect Differences**: Recognize and respect differences in background, perspectives, and goals. Tailor your mentoring approach to meet the individual needs of your mentee. Respecting differences between you and your mentee is essential for a successful mentor–mentee relationship. Encourage honest conversations. Discuss expectations, preferences, and any potential conflicts

openly. Recognize that differences in backgrounds, experiences, and perspectives enrich the relationship. Understand their point of view and show empathy. Avoid judgment or assumptions. Adapt your mentoring style to suit their needs. Be open to different learning styles and communication preferences.

13. **Seek Feedback**: Don't hesitate to ask for feedback from your mentee about your mentoring style and how you can better support them. Continuous improvement is valuable for both mentor and mentee. Asking for feedback from your mentee is essential for continuous improvement. Make it an ongoing process rather than a one-time event. Regularly check in with your mentee to gather insights. Ask directly for feedback. Be specific about what you'd like to know. For example, inquire about areas of strength and two aspects where you can improve. Show gratitude and respect when receiving feedback. Reflect on the lessons learned and take action to enhance your mentoring skills. Remember, feedback helps you grow as a mentor!
14. **End the Relationship Gracefully**: When the mentorship has achieved its goals or reached a natural conclusion, wrap up the relationship with gratitude and acknowledgment of the progress made. Ending a mentoring relationship gracefully is important. Here are some steps to consider:

    - **Reflect**: Evaluate the overall experience. Consider how it influenced your growth and learning.
    - **Open Communication**: Schedule a meeting with your mentor. Be transparent about your current view of the relationship and any changes in your situation.
    - **Closure and Gratitude**: Express gratitude for their time and contribution. Discuss future steps and how you plan to stay in touch.
    - **Celebrate Success**: Acknowledge achievements and part on a positive note.

Remember, ending a mentorship doesn't burn bridges—it's a natural part of the mentoring cycle.

Conclusion

Remember that a mentoring relationship is a partnership, and our active participation and commitment are crucial to its success. Being a good mentee not only benefits our own development but also contributes to a positive and productive mentoring experience for both you and our mentor. When the time comes, being a good mentor is about fostering the growth and development of our mentee while respecting their individuality and needs. It's a two-way relationship that can be enriching for both parties involved. It's easy to see how successful mentoring relationships incorporate aspects of all we've discussed in the previous chapters and how these core concepts are foundational to our development as physician leaders.

Take-Home Points

- Cultivating mentoring relationships is crucial for physician leaders to develop their careers and personal growth.
- Throughout our careers, we will be both mentor and mentee and need to learn how to perform in each role.
- Recognizing the importance of mentorship to our team members is crucial to their development and the success of our teams.

Reference

1. UCSF mentoring toolkit for forms, worksheets, and further reading

Chapter 10
Academic Appointment and Promotions

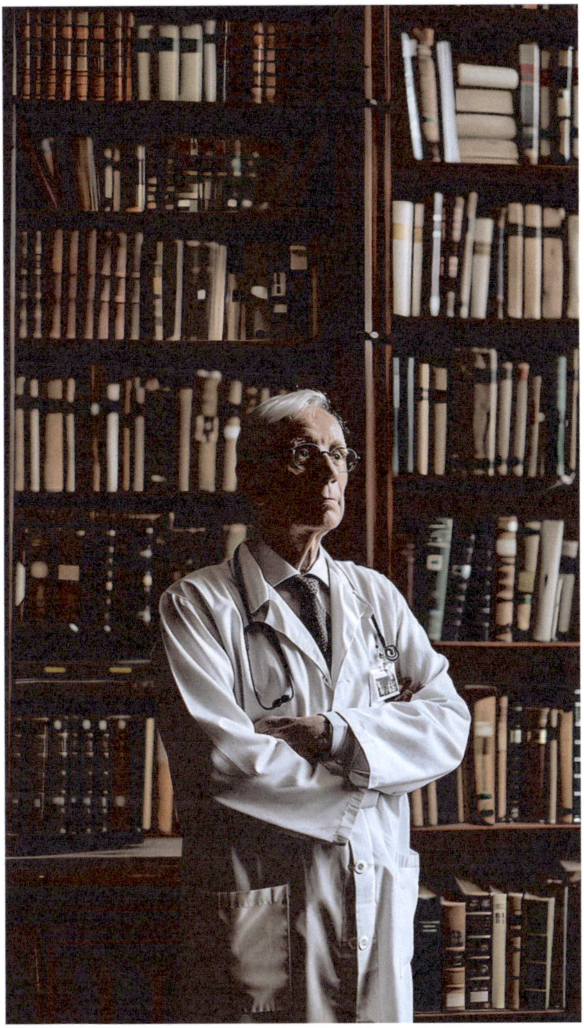

A. Djamali et al., *Emerging Leaders in Academic Medicine*,
https://doi.org/10.1007/978-3-031-80358-1_10

Case Presentation

Dr. Banks is a female physician clinical assistant professor at an academic medical center who contacted me to discuss the academic appointment process. As a promotion coordinator, I am available as a resource to all faculty at all stages of their career, and this is my first time interacting with Dr. Banks in this context.

Reviewing Dr. Banks's curriculum vitae in preparation for our meeting showed that she entered medicine following an undergraduate concentration in the biological sciences, during which time she was active in public health advocacy and peer tutoring programs. During medical school, she successfully completed research projects resulting in two publications (one as first author). As a faculty member at our institution, Dr. Banks participates in multiple, but varied, committee roles within her division; she engages in the clinical education of trainees but has not kept up documentation of this work on her CV; and she lists multiple invited academic presentations, but it is unclear if these were talks, abstracts, or poster presentations. The extent and description of her clinical work and roles is also difficult to discern from her CV.

Dr. Banks is now late in her third year of employment. She begins our meeting by telling me that while she completed a session on academic promotion during onboarding training when first hired, given how far away it seemed at that time, she did not pay much attention to the session. She has also received some mentoring and guidance from her division director in terms of handling her clinical practice and engaging with students but did not receive any direction about how to select academic commitments with an eye toward shaping her career and preparing for promotion. Dr. Banks further explains that with everything she has going on professionally and personally, she has rarely had time to even think about her promotion, let alone sit down to work on any required materials. Dr. Banks is aware that detailed information about the process and templates for documents are available online. However, Dr. Banks feels overwhelmed and anxious due to the scope of required materials, uncertainty of why academic promotion matters to a clinician, and lack of direction provided by her division and department. She is now discouraged, questioning whether to pursue promotion at all.

Introduction

While Dr. Banks's journey to and through promotion is unique, the feelings she experienced are hardly so. Junior faculty may receive limited mentorship and protected time to work on promotion, and the complex and lengthy promotion process lends itself to opacity and gatekeeping. However, while individual requirements vary from institution to institution, enough commonalities exist that it is possible to create a plan to put yourself in the strongest possible position for promotion when beginning a career in academic medicine.

Academic Promotion

Getting Started (Fig. 10.1)

In general, the entry-level academic appointment is at the rank of instructor, progressing to assistant professor, associate professor, and professor. In general, this ranking order is applicable in all North American schools (medicine or not). The criteria for promotion are local recognition (assistant professor), regional recognition (associate professor), and national/internal recognition (full professor). There is, in general, a 5-year requirement between promotion requests. The promotion application, review, and selection are an arduous and rigorous process that includes external referees and committees and takes about 6 months (used to be much longer).

Why Pursue Academic Promotion?

This may not be a question many people think about, as promotion is a requirement at most academic medical centers, and current ACGME guidelines expect faculty members who teach in GME programs to hold appropriate academic appointments.[1] Outside of this, academic promotion reflects a significant milestone of professional accomplishment and may be associated with higher income or leadership positions in national organizations or grant applications.

Time in rank	Clinical service	Teaching	Research	Professionalism/level of reputation (local, regional, national, international?)	Number oflLetters (external/internal)	CV–format required?	Required supplemental materials?

Fig. 10.1 Worksheet to complete. When reviewing your department/institution guidelines and requirements for promotion, complete the below chart as a quick reference sheet for the years leading up to promotion. Add any information that will be helpful for you. Items could include numbers of years/letters needed, documentation required for key areas of promotion, and supplemental materials (amount and type)

[1] Common Program Requirements (acgme.org)

Understanding Your Institution's Culture, Policies, and Procedures

Upon joining your institution, if you are not given a copy of policies and procedures on academic appointments and promotions, request one or obtain a copy from the institution's website. Most will be able to be found under the "Appointments and Promotions" tab of the Faculty Affair's website. The format and contents of guidelines will vary from institution to institution, but each will cover the same basic information (Table 10.1):

Table 10.1 General requirements

Clinical track—areas of evaluation	
Primary mission	Clinical care; noteworthy contribution to education of learners, support of the enterprise, research and discovery
Focus for promotion	Reputation and productivity, teaching excellence, contributions to research, scholarship and impact, enterprise leadership; specific criteria determined by the department and approved by TUSM/Dean's Office
Secondary objectives	Metrics reflecting clinical care quality (wide local referral base; participation in clinical programs that are locally or regionally distinctive); research productivity, education of learners, publications, grant funding
Minimum years to promotion	5 years is standard for nontenure track clinical faculty (some institutions have slightly different timelines)
Scholarship effort	Scholarship required; effort varies per focus; remember broad definition of scholarship beyond publications
Research funding	Supportive but not required
Professionalism	Required
Clinician-educator—areas of evaluation	
Primary mission	Clinical care; noteworthy contribution to education of learners, support of the enterprise, research and discovery
Focus for promotion	Teaching impact and excellence
Secondary objectives	Metrics reflecting clinical care quality (wide local referral base; participation in clinical programs that are locally or regionally distinctive); research productivity, education of learners, publications, grant funding
Minimum years to promotion	5 years is standard for nontenure track clinical faculty (some institutions have slightly different timelines)
Scholarship effort	Scholarship required; remember broad definition of scholarship beyond publications
Research funding	Supportive but not required
Professionalism	Required

(continued)

Table 10.1 (continued)

Tenure—areas of evaluation	
Primary mission	Academic output in all areas: clinical care and reputation; noteworthy contribution to education of learners and investigation
Focus for promotion	National reputation and sustained academic productivity, teaching excellence, contributions to research, high-impact scholarship, enterprise leadership, clinical reputation and impact
Secondary objectives	Metrics reflecting clinical care quality (wide local referral base; participation in clinical programs that are locally or regionally distinctive)
Minimum years to promotion	5 years is standard for nontenure track clinical faculty (some institutions have slightly different timelines)
Scholarship effort	Scholarship required, both publications and examples under newer, broader definitions
Research funding	Required
Professionalism	Required

Research—areas of evaluation	
Primary mission	Research and discovery; noteworthy contributions to education of learners; support of the enterprise
Focus for promotion	Contributions to research, scholarship and impact, securing funding
Secondary objectives	Noteworthy contributions to education
Minimum years to promotion	5 years is standard for nontenure track clinical faculty (some institutions have slightly different timelines)
Scholarship effort	Required
Research funding	Required
Professionalism	Required

- **Academic Tracks for Physicians**: In general, one's academic track is based on the alignment between institutional priorities in the areas of patient care, education, and research, and your accomplishments, skills, and interest in each area. Academic tracks may be specifically described in the job description when posted and therefore included as part of the initial offer letter. Alternatively, it can be established after hiring. In general, academic tracks follow this type of distribution:
  - Clinical track
  - Clinician-educator track
  - Tenure/unmodified track
  - Research track

It is important to have a good understanding of the expectations for appointment and promotion on each track, ideally before you are hired. When considering which track to pursue, always keep in mind that you strive for a fulfilling personal and professional life while building your career.

- *Clinical Track*: If you are an assistant professor on the clinical track (clinical assistant professor), most of your time will be devoted to patient care. This would represent anywhere between 32 and 38 hours of patient contact per week. You will not have unlimited access to medical residents, but you will be involved with the education of undergraduate and postgraduate trainees, including medical students and residents. The timeline and expectations for academic promotion are not as rigorous as the other tracks. This track is ideal if you greatly appreciate patient care in an academic setting but don't want to be heavily involved in research and education beyond citizenship expectations.

- *Clinical-Educator Track*: This track would be a good fit if you are a passionate educator and have an established percent of your FTE dedicated to teaching. Usually, a clinical-educator track faculty member would have anywhere between 5% and 20% nonclinical time to focus on education, research, innovation, and quality improvement projects. You would have a greater exposure to learners, primarily medical students, residents, and fellows. Teaching in an academic medical center is considered a privilege and comes with significant responsibility related to your impact and influence on the future of your students/learners. You should be ready to receive feedback from learners and strive for meritocracy among your peers. The timeline and expectations for academic promotion are described below and are more rigorous than the clinical track. The clinical-educator track is ideal if you greatly appreciate patient care in an academic setting but don't want to be heavily involved in research.
- *Tenure/Unmodified Track*: A highly prestigious pathway, which requires the highest level of achievement as a "triple threat" in clinical, research, and teaching settings. In general, you would have up to 75% protected time to pursue your academic work. This means your recruitment would require extramural funding, in general, in the form of mentored-career development grants from the NIH or national societies. You should consider this highly competitive track if you feel ready to take on "publish or perish," since promotion on the tenure track requires that you demonstrate independence from your primary mentor after 5 years, with additional extramural funding and, in general, more than 10 first- or last-author quality papers.
- *Research Track*: The research track is reserved for faculty who direct nearly all their professional effort to investigation and (almost always) do not carry out clinical activities. They should hold promise to evolve into independent investigators. Demonstration of ongoing laboratory or clinical research is an important consideration for appointment; publication of substantial original studies is required. A consistent funding record and publication of original investigations in which the candidate has played a leading role (as determined by first or last authorship) are key criteria for judging excellence in investigation.
- **Requirements for Associate Professor and Professor Ranks**: As this book is for junior faculty, the promotion discussion will focus on promotion to the rank of associate professor. What is said here also pertains to the general process of preparing for promotion to professor; however, the expectations for that rank are higher, and the process is generally more time-consuming.
  - Professional Recognition: Building a regional or national reputation can seem daunting in consideration of the amount of time devoted to patient care.

However, there are ways to incrementally work toward this and tackle it proactively, as the deadline for promotion is, in general, longer than on the tenure/unmodified track. When considering how to establish and build your reputation, it is important to choose with intention; quantity is good, but a sustained area of focus helps demonstrate expertise and reputation. For the associate professor level, a local and regional reputation is required. National or international is great, but not often expected or required until professor. Reputation can be supported by invited presentations, visiting professorships, membership in professional societies, positions on editorial boards, or ad hoc reviewer positions for journals.

Invited Presentations and Visiting Professorships: Ask about opportunities to present at division or department grand rounds at your institution. Mentors or colleagues from residency or fellowship can also be connections to getting invitations to present at their institution. Ask your mentors to contact their colleagues to get you invited for talks at peer institutions. Some programs have informal exchange processes in place to support their junior faculty for regional or national presentations.
Professional Societies: There are a seemingly unending number of professional societies to choose from, and you may already be a member of some at this point in your career. These organizations help you become a member of a community of people with common interests and goals and can help support your professional development. In general, you will want to be a member of one or two societies in your area of subspecialty.
External Committee Service: Join committees as you are interested and get involved, either by volunteering yourself or by putting your name out there to be volunteered by division chief, teaching colleagues, or clinical peers. Clinical committees can be of any nature; however, it is important to join committees that relate to your area of clinical expertise or interest, as it will help build your reputation in the area, and leadership positions on such committees can support reputation in the field. Members of these committees may be considered as external referees to write letters of recommendation for your promotion later.
Editorial Boards and/or Ad Hoc Reviewer: Selection or invitation for editorial boards and/or ad hoc reviewers for journals is important and often considered separately from one's external committee service. Not only do these roles offer invaluable learning experiences about the publication and editorial process, but they also allow a candidate a way to keep up with current literature, increase visibility with the field, and establish connections with potential collaborators.

– Scholarship/Publications: There is no magic rule for the number of publications required for promotion to associate professor, as they differ per track and institution. For example, while you may not need to publish a single paper for promotion on the clinical track at some institutions, even ten first- and last-author manuscripts may not be sufficient for promotion on the tenure track at a top-tier institution. Three general points are worth considering. First, you need to know the requirements for promotion at your institution. Next, you need to understand the guidelines of authorship by reviewing the International Committee of Medical Journal Editors (ICMJE) guidelines.[2] Discuss authorship at early stages before drafting the paper. This will avoid hard feelings and misunderstandings. First-author papers demonstrate your ability to think critically and complete the rigorous and laborious tasks of analyzing, synthesizing, writing, and teamwork. Last-author papers demonstrate your independence, leadership, and mentorship skills. Middle-author papers determine your ability to collaborate and cooperate. A blend of first-, middle-, and last-author papers looks good on any CV. The third and last point about scholarship and publications is to understand the impact of your work. With the explosion of online journals, it may be easier to publish low-quality work. On the other hand, not all papers need to be published in the *New England Journal of Medicine*, *Nature*, or *Science*. Online tools, including Impact Factor, H-Index, and Citation Report,[3] allow you to assess the quality of your published manuscript and/or destination journal. Despite their limitations, these tools provide a global understanding of the impact of your work. For example, an H-index greater than 12 is, in general, accepted by most institutions for promotion to associate professor.

- Service/Citizenship: Generally considered committee work performed within the larger institution of one's employment. This can be at the departmental-, hospital-, school-, university/institution-wide level. For associate professors, service at the departmental, hospital, and school levels is frequently sufficient. Another aspect of service to consider is the level of role one performs in the group. A majority of memberships with a few leadership/advanced roles is frequently enough to meet the service requirement at the associate professor level; however, given the time and effort it often takes to achieve chair/leadership roles, one should consider this progression plan while a junior faculty member.
- Clinical Scope: Most institutions require a strong local/regional referral base for the associate professor rank. A national base would be considered exceptional.
- Research: Academic physicians who are not focused on research, it is important to remember that research can be any of the following: bench, clinical, translational, epidemiological/biostatistical, health services, or QI/QA projects.
- Teaching: Amount and level will vary depending on whether or not education is the candidate's primary area of focus. However, medical student education, resident instruction, classroom and clinical, and mentoring are all teaching activities that should be recorded.

- **Minimum Years to Promotion/Time in Rank**: Most institutions will require a candidate be in rank (i.e., serving as an assistant professor or associate professor) for a set amount of time before being eligible for consideration for promotion.

---

[2] ICMJE | Recommendations | Defining the Role of Authors and Contributors

[3] Clarivate

Generally, this is 5 years at most institutions; however, many allow for candidates to start the process before that time or allow a window of 4–6 years in rank. This information will be clearly stated in departmental and/or institutional guidelines. Depending on the track, you may be able to retire as a clinical assistant professor, while you may have to find another job if you don't get promoted to associate professor and granted tenure track after 6 years.

- **Yes to No Ratio!** How often should you say "yes" and how often should you say "no" to opportunities as you start your academic career? The yes/no ratio for an enthusiastic junior faculty member is, in general, significantly greater than 1, which is understandable. You want to be promoted, you are learning the lay of the land, and you don't want to disappoint your more experienced, senior colleagues. Conversely, the ratio may be less than 1 for senior faculty members. This is because they are more experienced, differentiated, and, in general, successful. So, they can afford turning down opportunities. Academic promotion is an incredible personal and professional milestone. To achieve this goal, sacrifices need to be made. But you don't want to burn out early on in your career. That is why it is important to have personal and professional priorities (even if you must reevaluate them frequently) and a mentor or mentoring committee to guide you toward a yes/no ratio that is compatible with those priorities.

Components of the Dossier

- **Documenting Activity: CV**

- "If you do it, document it." Best practice is to schedule a monthly (or even weekly, if you can) appointment on your calendar to update your CV with all relevant details as close to the time of the event as possible. Looking back 5 years after the fact when preparing for promotion and having to fill in entries from memories or whatever records you may have kept is time-consuming and can even be a limiting factor in some clinicians pursuing academic promotion. This is even more critical for those clinicians pursuing leadership opportunities, as they will have numerous trainings, positions, conferences, teaching activities, and publications to document.
- **Personal Statement**:
- The personal statement is your chance to show how you view your career to date and discuss the achievements you feel have made the most impact. This narrative framework ties these elements together and shows how you view your career holistically. The statement should provide context and your own take on the highlights of your career, rather than simply relisting what is stated on your CV. While the tone and structure can range from informal to very formal, you will be asked to address your:

  - Clinical/public health activities, any novel features of their clinical/public health work, and a summary of scholarly activity

  - Teaching contributions, philosophy, and novel work in the field
  - Institutional leadership role or leadership service on national committees/organizations

- **Letter Writers**
- Securing referee letters is often the most difficult part of the promotion process. However, there are some things to keep in mind that can help lessen anxiety around this step. You will be asked to provide names of potential referees in two categories: internal colleagues with whom you work and external/arms-length ones with whom you have no connection. Regardless of the internal/external category, the letters should be from people who are in a position to judge the candidate's accomplishments, reputation, and worthiness for promotion. It is also crucial to note that letters can only be provided by individuals who are at or above the rank you are being considered for.
- Some additional considerations for external, independent letter writers:
  - External referee letters should be provided by people who are considered to be external and independent from the candidate. It is important to include letters from people who can give an informed opinion that is not influenced by a present or prior relationships.
  - They cannot be current or former peers, research or scholarly partners, people you have published with, people from inside your institution/its system, former mentors or mentees, students, or close clinical associates.
  - They can be from people who are familiar with your work or reputation, people you have loosely served with on a national committee, or people who have invited you to speak at their program or conference.

- **Supporting/Supplemental Documentation**
- Often institutions ask for (can be required or optional) additional, supplemental materials to support one's application for promotion. This can be
  - **Teaching Portfolio**: Format and exact requirements will vary, but like the CV, keeping and updating a document of all teaching work will be of great help when promotion time comes. If a template is available online from your institution, you could use that from the beginning, but any system that allows you to track date of teaching activity, location/type (clinical vs. classroom), level of trainee, and number of students will be a huge help when preparing materials for promotion.
  - **Student Evaluations**: Although there are concerns with bias in course evaluations, they can still be useful in demonstrating positive learner impact. Quotes including specifics of the impact an instructor made or specifics about their teaching that were particularly good are strong supporting materials.
  - **Documentation of Clinical Excellence**: Like course evaluations, patient evaluations can show bias; however, just like student evaluations, they can also be strong supporting evidence showing clinical excellence and impact (notes from grateful patients would also fall under this grouping). Depending

on the specifics of clinical practice, patient panel information, volumes, before and after a provider arrived/assumed a patient group, etc. can be strong evidence in support of clinical impact.

- **Publications**: Many institutions are moving away from requiring publication reprints in the promotion dossier; however, some may still ask for the most significant or most representative publications that a candidate has written. If full prints are not required, this is often indicated on the CV by marking publications the candidate wishes to highlight.

Conclusion

While there are many parts to the academic promotion process, there is no need for the process to be a mystery. Reviewing and understanding institutional promotion guidelines early in one's career can alleviate the sense of unknown that can come with such an important career event and allow the candidate to know what will be required and to document those items in real time. Although it may remain a time of anxiety and nerves, it is entirely possible to demystify the promotion process and break it down into a series of manageable steps.

Take-Home Points

- *Plan*: Obtain a copy of promotion guidelines and note requirements. Consider your main clinical and academic interests. Find yourself a mentor or mentoring committee. Mentorship is a critical component of academic growth. We all mentor and need mentors, regardless of our academic rank. A special chapter in this book is assigned to this topic.
- *Participate*: Teach, serve on committees, participate in research, and engage with the medical community in a way that supports your interests and aligns with your larger career plan and area(s) of expertise.
- *Document*: If you do it, document it. Set a calendar appointment at regular intervals to update the CV, teaching documentation, information about research funding, publications, and invited presentations.

Index

A. Djamali et al., *Emerging Leaders in Academic Medicine*,
https://doi.org/10.1007/978-3-031-80358-1

MIX
Papier aus verantwortungsvollen Quellen
Paper from responsible sources
FSC® C105338
FSC
www.fsc.org

If you have any concerns about our products,
you can contact us on
ProductSafety@springernature.com

In case Publisher is established outside the EU,
the EU authorized representative is:
Springer Nature Customer Service Center GmbH
Europaplatz 3, 69115 Heidelberg, Germany

Printed by Libri Plureos GmbH
in Hamburg, Germany